Nursing Theories

Hesook Suzie Kim, PhD, RN, is Professor of Nursing at the University of Rhode Island and Professor II at the Institute of Nursing Science, Faculty of Medicine, University of Oslo in Norway since 1992. She was the Dean of the College of Nursing, University of Rhode Island from 1983 to 1988 and has been teaching at the University since 1973. Her PhD is in sociology from Brown University, Providence, Rhode Island. She has been published widely in the areas of nursing epistemology, theory development in nursing, the nature of nursing practice, and collaborative decision making in nursing practice as well as in various areas of clinical nursing research. She is the author of a seminal book on the metaparadigm of nursing published in 1983, *The Nature of Theoretical Thinking in Nursing.* The revised edition is in press (Springer, 2000). She is the co-author of two chapters on critical philosophy in *In Search of Nursing Science* edited by Omery, Kasper, and Page (1995) and published in collaboration with Inger Margrethe Holter. She has been instrumental in bringing about the 5-year series on *Knowledge Development Symposia* held in Newport, Rhode Island from 1990 to 1994. It examined the linkages among philosophy, theory development, method, and practice as related to knowledge development in nursing.

Ingrid Kollak, PhD, is Professor of Nursing Science at Alice-Salomon University of Applied Sciences in Berlin, Germany. She received her PhD in philology from Universität Essen, Germany. Her areas of specialization are history of nursing and medicine, educational systems, and nursing theory. She is the author of *Literatur und Hypnose. Der Mesmerismus und sein Einfluß auf die Literatur des 19. Jahrhunderts* (Frankfurt/New York, 1997) and *Innovative Entwicklungen im Gesundheitswesen und ihre Konsequenzen für die Kompetenzentwicklung von Führungskräften und Mitarbeitern* (Berlin, 1998). She is the co-author of *Gesundheitsvorsorge bei Menschen mit Diabetes mellitus* (Stuttgart, 1998, with Barbara Senftleben) and *Pflege verwirrter alter Menschen* (Stuttgart, 1998, with Eva Schmitt). She has co-edited the volumes *Pflege-Ausbildung im Gespräch. Ein internationaler Vergleich* (Frankfurt, 1998, with Angelika Pillen) and *Pflegediagnosen: was leisten sie, was leisten sie nicht?* (Frankfurt, 1999, with Margret Georg).

Nursing Theories

Conceptual and Philosophical Foundations

Hesook Suzie Kim, PhD, RN
Ingrid Kollak, PhD
Editors

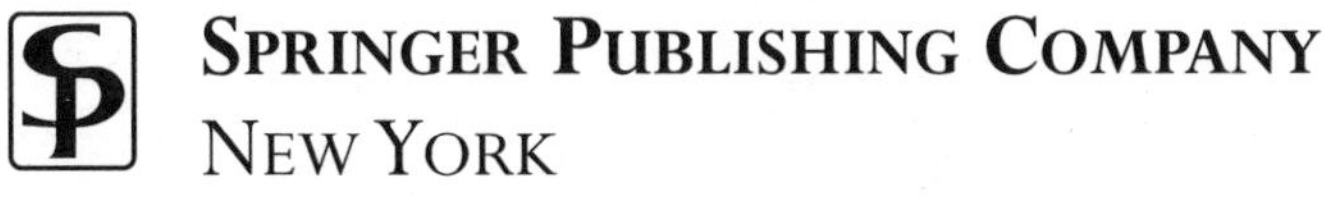
SPRINGER PUBLISHING COMPANY
NEW YORK

Springer Publishing Company, Inc.
536 Broadway
New York, NY 10012-3955

Acquisitions Editor: Ruth Chasek
Production Editor: J. Hurkin-Torres
Cover design by James Scotto-Lavino

99 00 01 02 03 / 5 4 3 2 1

Library of Congress Cataloging-in-Publication Data

Nursing theories : conceptual and philosophical foundations / Hesook Suzie Kim and Ingrid Kollak, editors.
p. cm.
Includes bibliographical references and index.
ISBN 0-8261-1287-0 (hardcover)
1. Nursing—Philosophy. I. Kim, Hesook Suzie. II. Kollak, Ingrid.
[DNLM: 1. Nursing Theory. 2. Models, Nursing. 3. Philosophy, Nursing. WY 86 N97374 1999]
RT84.5.N8795 1999
610.73'01—dc21
DNLM/DLC
for Library of Congress 99-27969
CIP

Printed in the United States of America

Contents

Contributors

Friedrich Balke, PhD, holds a PhD in philosophy from Ruhr-Universität Bochum and is an academic coordinator of the postgraduate research school at the University of Siegen in Germany. He has published widely on political philosophy, social and cultural theory, and contemporary French philosophy.

May Solveig Fagermoen, PhD, RN, is an Associate Professor at the Institute of Nursing Science at University of Oslo in Norway and is currently the Director of the Institute. She received her basic nursing education from Aker School of Nursing, and Nurse Teacher's degree from the Norwegian School of Advanced Studies in Nursing. She holds an MA in nursing from the University of Washington School of Nursing in Seattle, Washington, and a PhD in nursing from University of Rhode Island, Kingston, Rhode Island. She has published two books on teaching and learning in nursing.

Jacqueline D. Fortin, DNSc, RN, is an Associate Professor of nursing at the University of Rhode Island. She received a BS in nursing from the University of Rhode Island, an MS in nursing from Boston College, and a DNSc degree from Boston University. She has been a faculty member at the University of Rhode Island since 1974. For the past 14 years she has taught mainly in the College of Nursing's doctoral program and until recently was the coordinator for the Advanced Practice in Critical Care Nursing in the College's Master's program. In addition to her teaching, she has been involved in an ongoing program of funded clinical research and publication, primarily in the area of postoperative pain.

Jens Friebe, Dr. rer. Soc., is currently a head of training and in-service training for nursing occupations at the vocational training center of the German Trades Union under the umbrella organization, Berufsfortbildungswerk des Deutschen Gewerkschaftsbundes in Bochum, Germany. He is a state-registered nurse in the care for the elderly, and holds both a diploma that is equivalent to a Master's degree and a doctorate in social sciences. He has an extensive nursing experience in gerontological and psychiatric nursing, and has published in the areas of intercultural gerontology, networking in nursing, and curriculum development.

Penny Powers, PhD, RN, is Associate Professor and Department head for South Dakota State University College of Nursing in Rapid City, South Dakota. She earned her PhD in nursing from the University of Washington, Seattle, Washington. She has worked as a medical/surgical nurse in Canada and is also licensed in the United States. She writes about nursing research methodology and is editor of a book about discourse analysis which will be published by Sage in 1999.

Donna Schwartz-Barcott, PhD, RN, is a Professor and Director of Graduate Studies in nursing in the College of Nursing at the University of Rhode Island, Kingston, Rhode Island. She holds a PhD in anthropology from the University of North Carolina. She teaches courses in knowledge development in the client domain and inductive approaches to theory development in the doctoral program. She and Dr. Kim developed the Hybrid Model of Concept Development to enhance the theoretical and empirical grounding of core concepts in nursing, which was published in *Concept Development in Nursing: Approaches and Applications* edited by Rodgers and Knafl (1993). She has co-authored several articles dealing with a variety of fieldwork approaches (e.g., ethnography and action research) to inductive theory development, including some newer strategies for enhancing the linkage between practice and theory development.

Charlotte Uzarewicz, Dr. disc. pol., is Professor of Nursing Science and Nursing Management at the Confessional (Protestant) University of Applied Science (Evangelische Fachhochschule Berlin) in Berlin, Germany. She is a nurse, social/cultural anthropologist with an MA degree in anthropology, and a sociologist with a doctorate in political science. Her areas of research are history of science, racism, theories of culture and identity, transcultural nursing, and theories of the body.

Susanne Wied, MA, is a nurse, a nurse-teacher, and a Gordon-Communications trainer. She holds a Master's degree in nursing education (Diplom-Pflegepädagogin) from Humboldt-Universität in Berlin. She teaches nursing theories and nursing ethics at Institute for Nursing and Communication (Institut für Pflege und Kommunikation) in Berlin, Germany, and is interested in communication-training and visual perception research. She has a book in press: *Das Phänomen der Farbe und ihrer Wahrnehmung* to be published by Eicanos Verlag in Germany.

ABOUT THE TRANSLATORS

This book has been written as a collaboration of U.S., German, and Norwegian nurses. The German chapters were translated into English by the following individuals:

Ellen M. Klein received a BA in German and Linguistics from the University of Michigan at Ann Arbor and a MA in German Linguistics from the Free University of Berlin.

Gerald Nixon teaches translation and essay writing at Berlin's Free University. He received a BA in the study of Modern Languages in England.

Preface

The idea for this book came about when we were together in Berlin in the summer of 1996. Ingrid had been talking with a German publisher who was interested in publishing a book about nursing theories. This led us to discussing the current situation in the discipline of nursing both in the United States and in Europe regarding theory development and theoretical discourse. We both felt that there is a great need to have a theory book that was not just elaborating on contents of nursing theories, but that examined the conceptual and philosophical ideas behind nursing theories. Such a book, we thought, could assist advanced students in nursing to comprehend nursing's major theoretical ideas from foundational issues pertaining to theory development and relationship to nursing practice.

The intention of this book is a systematic, analytical treatise of nursing's major theoretical work through in-depth analyses of conceptual and philosophical ideas underpinning nursing theories and theoretical frameworks. It is not a survey of nursing theories, or an evaluation of nursing theories in terms of their theoretical structures and contents. However, readers will gain a deeper understanding of nursing theories through examining them in their conceptual and philosophical contexts. No nursing theory has been developed in a vacuum—each has rich and varied roots in Western conceptual and philosophical traditions, and this book allows readers to step back and view this larger picture. All of the themes we have selected for inclusion in this book are familiar to students of nursing, and may evoke different conceptual pictures for them. We believe this conceptual approach makes the book especially rich and interesting as well as challenging.

We hope that this book will be used as a companion to the original theoretical works for better understanding of not only the theories themselves but also essential questions about nursing theory development, such as how different conceptual and philosophical perspectives influence theoretical approaches to study key phenomena in nursing. We think this book initiates a third tier in the exposition of theoretical nursing: the first being the original theories proposed and advanced by various authors, the second tier focusing on analysis and evaluation of nursing's conceptual frameworks and theories. This third tier focuses on the analysis of concepts and issues forming the foundation of nursing theories' orientations and perspectives. This will, we hope, add to a comprehensive study of nursing's theoretical works.

The idea in the beginning was to work on such a book to be published in German with the contributions by both American- and German-speaking scholars in nursing. But as we got into the actual development of the outline and preparation of the manuscript, it became apparent to us that there would be great merit and excitement in publishing the book both in German and English concurrently. While it is quite true that European nurses and nursing scholars are exposed widely to theoretical work published in English, American readers have not had many opportunities to read analytical work regarding nursing theory written by German-speaking scholars, except for a limited number of journal articles published in English. In this age of globalism and multiculturalism, we find it exciting to present views and studies of nursing's theoretical issues by scholars not only with different philosophical orientations but also with different linguistic, cultural, and academic backgrounds. We have contributions from four American authors, one Norwegian scholar whose advanced degrees are from the United States, and five German authors. The contributors have done remarkable feats of pulling together sources of information and knowledge that undergird each theme and at the same time remaining utterly critical and analytical in their expositions. We are sure all contributors would agree with us that the intent of the book is to raise critical questions fundamental to advancing nursing's theoretical work than to provide definitive answers about what is good or bad about nursing theories.

As with any edited book, it is quite amazing how one can achieve diversity in characteristics as we find in the chapters included in this book. Without the contributors' insights and knowledge as well as their diligence and perseverance, this book would not have materialized. We need also to acknowledge an important contribution made by the translators who translated German manuscripts into English for the American publication, and those who translated English manuscripts into German for the German publication. We would not have a comprehensible work without their sensitivity and understanding regarding terms as used in nursing and philosophy. We are also grateful for the support of our American editor, Ruth Chasek at Springer, and our German editor, Klaus Reinhardt at Huber Verlag.

Hesook Suzie Kim
Exeter, Rhode Island

Ingrid Kollak
Berlin, Germany

1

Introduction

Hesook Suzie Kim

Nursing's theoretical knowledge has a rich heritage in its development dating back to the writings of Florence Nightingale and emanating from the work of many nursing scholars of the past three decades. Although there is a continuing debate as to whether nursing theories as they exist presently are mature enough or rigorously developed, nursing theories, large and small, have become the cornerstone for understanding and guiding nursing practice in the current decade. However, there are many questions about nursing theories and their contents that trouble students of nursing, whether they are undergraduate or graduate students or practicing nurses.

One of the major difficulties voiced by many is related to the presence of numerous nursing theories, all of which claim to have answers to nursing questions and provide guidance to nursing practice. Although nursing theories in general are presented with the supposition that they are oriented to describing and explaining nursing's concerns, each is based on assumptions, philosophies, values, perspectives, and scope that are somewhat unique. Different foundational ideas, both conceptual and philosophical, orient nursing theories to describe and explain the phenomena of concern to nursing in diverse ways. While nursing theories in general are not presented with coherence among the theories' components, precision in conceptualization, and logic in structure, it is not too difficult to extract the theories' perspectives and assumptions that enlighten us about their orientations regarding how nursing phenomena are treated theoretically.

Many books written about nursing theories contain categorization of nursing theories into different sorts. For example, Meleis (1996) categorizes them having systems, holistic, adaptation, and behavioral orientations; and puts them into theories on nursing clients, on human being-environment interactions, on interactions, and on nursing therapeutics. On the other hand, Parse (1987) treats five nursing theoretical models in terms of the totality and simultaneity paradigms. Obviously, different nursing theories have been developed with various conceptual and philosophical orientations, which usually lay foundations for the ways theorists view humans, human life, human relations, or practice. Theoretical assumptions undergirding theories stem from differing conceptual and philosophical orientations, and they have intimate connections to theories' substantive contents.

We offer in this book expositions that analyze selected nursing theories' conceptual and philosophical foundations so that nursing theories are not only understood in terms of their contents but also from their foundational ideas. This is based on the belief that users of nursing theories for research, practice, or education must have an understanding and enlightenment about theories regarding not only what the theories aim to describe and explain, but also from what ontological and epistemological perspectives such theoretical descriptions and explanations are developed. This, we believe, can be done only through in-depth analyses of the foundational ideas, examined within broad contexts from which different conceptual and philosophical orientations originate.

THEMES AS THE BASES FOR THEORETICAL UNDERSTANDING

We have selected ten "themes" used as the basic orientations of nursing theories for examination in this book. These themes have become the major ideas which underlie nursing's theoretical development, and have provided different starting points for theory development and contents. Six of the themes are thought to have conceptual foci as their starting points, while three themes are primarily oriented to ontology of humans and one theme is specifically oriented to a philosophy of nursing.

A conceptual focus refers to a specific conceptualization of human aspects or nursing practice, and provides an angle of vision regarding the phenomena a theory is concerned with in offering understanding and explanation. In nursing theories, a conceptual focus often is a way of organizing our understanding of human phenomena. Conceptual themes have grounding in different domains of nursing, that is, in what Kim (1987) differentiated as the client domain, the client-nurse domain, the environment domain, and the practice domain.

Included in our analyses of nursing theories are the conceptual foci of *human needs* and *needs*, *adaptation*, and the *health/illness continuum* grounded in the client domain, which are concerned specifically with the conceptualization of clients and their nursing problems. These four themes are different conceptual orientations framing the phenomena in the client domain. Theories with their focus on these concepts view nursing clients primarily in terms of (a) in what state they are in with respect to what they need or require in order to sustain or grow (human needs focus), (b) how well they are in responding to forces that impinge on them (adaptation focus), and (c) how attribution of illness as risk and the conceptualization of health and illness as a continuum determine and influence the ways clients experience illness and patienthood.

In addition, *human interaction* as a theme in the client-nurse domain offers the bases from which nursing theories' orientations on client-nurse interaction are examined. Nursing has traditionally been interested in studying interaction as client-nurse interaction. This is viewed both as the medium through which nursing care is processed and as the mode with which nursing produces its therapeutic effectiveness. We also include analysis of the concept of *transculturality* in relation to nursing theories. The concept of transculturality is considered to have reference to the environment domain, as culture is an environmental context in relation to human health. The concept of transculturality is viewed as grounding humans who are nursing clients and nursing practice within cultural context.

Three themes, *holism*, *system*, and *existential phenomenology*, provide the analyses of nursing theories from their ontological beginnings. These are themes adopted by nursing theories as providing specific ontological perspectives regarding humans, human entity, and/or human experiences. The theme of *caring and humanism* provides a framework for examining nursing theory from the philosophy of nursing perspective.

Additionally, a critical examination of the development of nursing and nursing science from a socio-historical perspective provides an appreciation of the genesis of different conceptualizations and theories in nursing from the broader context of history.

A FRAMEWORK FOR THEORETICAL UNDERSTANDING

Many books are written about theories in nursing (for example, Meleis, 1996; Barnum, 1994; and Fitzpatrick & Whall, 1996). Most of these are oriented to analysis and critique of theories by adopting certain criteria for identifying theoretical assumptions, distinguishing contents, and evaluating the maturity, completeness, and logic of theory. In general, theories and theoretical frameworks are examined with respect to different components and aspects related to them. These are:

1. Theoretical perspectives—Provides insights to the theory's worldviews and angle of vision regarding the phenomena of interest from the conceptual, ontological, and epistemological orientations.
2. Basic assumptions and premises—Further illuminates the theory's orientations regarding how one is to understand and explain nursing phenomena.
3. Concepts and their definitions—Specifies major concepts used in the theory and their conceptualizations.
4. Theoretical structure and statements—Specifies the form of theory and its structure and the nature of theoretical statements developed for the theory.
5. Chronological order of progression—Provides an understanding regarding the order with which theory developed has progressed for a given theory.
6. Theorist(s) and major proponents—Provides insights into the theorist's scientific orientations that undergird the theory development.

Comprehending nursing theories requires multifaceted approaches beginning with a descriptive understanding of theories, which comes from a thorough reading of original work. From this initial understanding, one can move toward a critical understanding based on analysis and evaluation of a given theory in terms of what it proposes as well as the foundation from which its proposals originate. It further involves a strategic understanding through which one can gain an appreciation of the processes of theory development and the background under which a given theory has emerged. This can be done by analysis of a given theory's evolutionary progression and through an in-depth understanding of the philosophical and theoretical commitments of the major proponents of a given theory. Table 1.1 shows how such multilevel approaches may focus on different aspects of understanding nursing theories.

This book does not attempt to analyze nursing theories from all of these analytical schemas but is mainly oriented to the study of nursing theories from the analysis of foundational perspectives. The aim of this book is to provide a review and analysis of nursing theories that can add to the comprehension of theoretical work in nursing from a different approach from those adopted by major authors who focus on analyzing theories for their contents and logical structures. Our approach in this book is to examine nursing theories from the analysis of conceptual and

TABLE 1.1 Multifaceted Approach to Theoretical Comprehension

Types of analysis	Aspects of theory comprehension
Thorough reading	Understanding the language and structure of theory
Analysis of contents for metaparadigm orientation	Understanding the scope of theory
Analysis of theory structure	Understanding the theoretical precision and logic-in-use in terms of concepts and theoretical statements
Analysis of coherence among components	Understanding the coherence and organization among theoretical components
Analysis of foundational perspectives	Understanding the conceptual and philosophical orientations regarding the images of humans and nursing, conceptualization of key phenomena, and theoretical explanation
Analysis of theory progression	Understanding the theory development process
Study of theorist/major proponents	Understanding the theorist's perspectives and visions regarding theory development

philosophical perspectives that undergird nursing theories. The themes identified as the major conceptual and philosophical orientations are examined for their meaning, ontological orientations, and epistemological implications. Theories relevant to each of the themes are then examined and contrasted in the context of the theme's definitional, ontological, and epistemological discussions. Hence, the reviews are oriented to identifying and examining the foundational groundings with which the theories are developed. This level of studying theories will provide the readers with an appreciation of theories' perspectives and philosophical issues pertinent to theory development in nursing. This orientation has guided the analyses offered in the following chapters.

In chapter 2, the concept of adaptation is analyzed in its meanings used in relation to populations and species, and individuals. It furthermore addresses their implications for nursing's theoretical approaches regarding client phenomena. The concept of human needs is analyzed from a general analytic perspective in chapter 3 identifying some of the key need theories in nursing, while chapter 4 offers a discourse analysis of the current status of the concept of needs in nursing.

Issues of interaction and communication are analyzed in chapter 5 in relation to specific nursing theories dealing with client-nurse interaction.

In chapter 6, an analysis of the concepts of culture and transculturality is offered in relation to its meanings for clients and nursing practice, and are examined within the semantic field of the concepts and in relation to their epistemological potential.

In chapter 7, holism is investigated for its philosophical roots, identifying diverse orientations and multiple interpretations of this philosophy. It is then examined in relation to nursing theories, especially in terms of the theory of unitary human beings by Rogers, and implications of diverse holistic philosophies on nursing theory development. The concept and philosophy of system is examined in chapter 8, tracing it from the general systems orientation and social sciences. Nursing theories with a systems focus are then examined in their specific orientations within the concept of system. In chapter 9, the philosophy of existential phenomenology is described, tracing its philosophical roots in phenomenology and existentialism, and Parse's theory of human becoming is examined within the tenets of existential phenomenology. Chapter 10 offers an in-depth analysis of philosophies of humanism and caring and their implications for nursing theory development. The historical and philosophical origins of humanism and caring are traced and analyzed to depict and contrast how these philosophies are adopted in nursing theories. Chapter 11 deals with the conceptualizations of health/illness as a continuum and illness as risk and offers a postmodern critique that raises questions regarding the meanings of normality and abnormality and implications of illness concept as risk in developing theories about clients and health care in nursing.

In chapter 12, a broader question related to the development of nursing and nursing science is addressed from a sociohistorical perspective. This critique is offered from both diachronic and synchronic views, pointing out the necessity for nursing and nursing science to meet the challenges for growing autonomy in patient care. In chapter 13, a postscript is offered with an examination of the contexts of American and German nursing, nursing education, and nursing science.

REFERENCES

Barnum, B. J. S. (1994). *Nursing theory: Analysis, application, evaluation* (4th ed.). Philadelphia: Lippincott.

Fitzpatrick, J. J., & Whall, A. L. (1996). *Conceptual models of nursing: Analysis and application* (3rd ed.). Stamford, CT: Appleton & Lange.

Kim, H. S. (1987). Structuring the nursing knowledge system: A typology of four domains. *Scholarly Inquiry for Nursing Practice: An International Journal, 1,* 99–110.

Meleis, A. I. (1996). *Theoretical nursing: Development and progress* (3rd ed.). Philadelphia: Lippincott.
Parse, R. R. (1987). *Nursing science: Major paradigms, theories, and critiques.* Philadelphia: Saunders.

2

Adaptation as a Basic Conceptual Focus in Nursing Theories

Donna Schwartz-Barcott

Adaptation is a popular and long-standing term in nursing. It is used most frequently to capture a central concern of the discipline: an individual's adjustment to an illness, a disability, or health problem. It has been cited as a key term in the nursing literature since the mid-1950s, with the appearance of the first edition of the *Cumulative Index to Nursing and Allied Literature*. Since then, it has been used as a general subject heading to encompass the term in its most common dictionary meanings as (a) the act or process of adapting—as in adapting to a nursing home or (b) the state of being adapted—as in being physically or psychologically well adapted to diabetes. It also has been used to include the term in its form as an adjective, referring to one's ability to adapt. Hall's (1991) article on adaptability as a personal resource influencing one's health uses the term in this manner.

Over the last 30 years, the primary thrust in the nursing literature has been on adaptation as a process, whether that process be conscious or unconscious, that includes physiological, psychological, and sociocultural mechanisms and can be seen as a success or failure. The focus on adaptation as an outcome has been secondary, although it seems to be gaining attention, given the current emphasis in nursing on developing and measuring patient outcomes.

Although the term has been used overwhelmingly at the individual client level in nursing, it also has been employed at family and population levels as well as in the practice domain to address issues regarding the adaptability of nurses. For example, since the 1960s there has been a small but continually increasing interest in how parents and families adjust when a member of the family, particularly a child, is acutely or chronically ill or disabled. The relatively rare citations at the population level deal mainly with how communities adapt to changing health needs or how a minority group attempts to deal with health problems associated with migration. In the practice domain, the predominant interest has been in the problems nurses face as students (either national or international) and as employees, in transition from being students to professional nurses or from a traditional role into a new role (e.g., that of the nurse practitioner, operating room or home care nurse as well as the educator or administrator), or under new conditions (e.g., shift work) or difficult situations such as working with terminally ill patients.

As early as 1962, a small group of educators had begun to discuss and write about adaptation theory as a possible conceptual framework for nursing (Brown, 1963; Levine, 1966; Martin & Prange, 1962). They were looking for a conceptual framework that could be used to: (a) develop more integrated curriculum, (b) serve as a theoretical basis for nursing practice, and (c) provide clues for improvement of patient care.

It was the broad conception of human phenomena, the unifying view of human biological, psychological, and social functioning underlying adaptation theory and its potential for integrating knowledge from diverse disciplines that initially was so attractive and held such promise for nursing.

In the years that followed, nurses have drawn directly from the continuing development and refinement of various conceptualizations both from outside and within nursing. It is the conceptions underlying these efforts that will be the focus of the remainder of this chapter.

BEGINNING CONCEPTUALIZATIONS OF ADAPTATION: POPULATIONS ADAPTING

In its most general form, adaptation has been used in a broad range of disciplines (including biology, physiology, genetics, anthropology, sociology, and psychology, as well as nursing) to refer to the mechanisms or processes that act to maintain a living entity in balance with its environment. That entity might be the human species, a society, a group, or an individual organism—a human being. However, the earliest scientific interest in the concept almost always is linked to biology and to Darwin's efforts at describing the mechanisms involved in long-term evolutionary change at the species or population level (first in plants, then in animals, and finally in the human species) (Alland & McCay, 1973).

As a young naturalist, Darwin (1859) made a trip around the world on the now famous HMS Beagle. On the voyage, he accumulated a vast store of data and observed a wide range of species that seemed particularly well adapted to specific environmental niches. For example, on the Galapagos Islands, Darwin observed 13 species of finches that were apparently of common origin but had developed structural differences that suited them for a variety of niches. They differed in size and beak structure, depending on what they ate and whether they were ground or tree dwellers (Lerner, 1968). Darwin tried to describe, retrospectively, the process through which these changes in physical structure had occurred and how these were sustained across generations. Darwin went on to describe this process in terms of variability and natural selection. With the advent of population genetics in the 1930s, differential reproductive success provided the missing mechanism by which variability and natural selection resulted in transgenerational evolutionary change.

Thus, adaptation became closely aligned with the study of evolutionary change and survival. It was seen as a process by which a species interacted with and became fitted to its environment to obtain food, shelter, and protection from predation. Ultimately, this would ensure the biological survival of the species (*Encyclopedia of Sociology*, 1974). A basic assumption was that any living system exists within a given environment, and it must adapt to that environment to survive. In this context, adaptation is not a conscious, goal-directed activity. It is the result of the differential reproductive success of populations, which is determined by the conditions of the moment, not by ultimate desirability or by the remote future (Washburn & Lancaster, 1968). It is worth noting here, that in this context:

1. The process is based on a species or a population. It is the population, not an individual that evolves. Individuals are part of the process but survival is at the population or species level and not at the individual level.
2. The response is to environmental conditions; the population either moves into a new environment or something changes in the population or species in response to the environment.
3. Analytically, one starts with a population that is already adapted to its environment.
4. Survival over a long timeframe is the outcome of interest.

A major and enduring criticism of this theoretical work has been that the concept of adaptation is tautological, that is, whatever is there is considered adaptive. As Alland and McCay note (1973) this is illustrated in the supposedly "self-evident" characteristic of biological adaptation whereby "organisms are surviving because they are adapted and they are adapted because they are surviving" (p. 144). This confusion is not helped when different forms of the term adaptation are used to label both the process and its outcome.

ADAPTATION AND THE EVOLUTION OF SOCIETIES

Parallel developments took place in anthropology and sociology in the mid nineteenth century among scholars interested in the evolution of societies. These early developments are associated with the writings of the English philosopher Herbert Spencer (Harris, 1968). By the 1900s, a major focus of those interested in societal evolution was on identifying the cultural and social mechanisms (e.g., technological, organizational, and ideational) that enhanced a society's adjustment to conditions of existence and thus increased its chances of survival (Carneiro, 1973; Service, 1968). In this context, the notion of environment was broadened to include not only the natural environment but also the social environment, although the unit of adaptation was still at the population level, and the outcome was primarily on survival. This interest in societal adaptation and evolution has continued and currently can be seen in the works of scholars, including Carneiro (1973), Service (1968), Harris (1968), and McElroy and Townsend (1996) in anthropology and Parsons (1964), Eisenstadt (1968), and Lenski, Lenski, and Nolan (1995) in sociology.

Although adaptation is most frequently linked with evolutionary change, it has also been studied throughout this timeframe with regard to more short-term and nonevolutionary change. One would expect the type of adaptive mechanisms or processes involved with evolutionary change to be different from those dealing with short-term change. It was based on a concern for identifying and distinguishing between these processes that Alland and McCay (1973) suggested that "adaptation" be considered as the physiological response of organisms (e.g., a homeostatic response to short-term variations in the environment—such as adaptations to temperature change) and "transgenerational adaptation" be used as an outcome of the evolutionary process (p. 144).

ADAPTATION AT THE INDIVIDUAL LEVEL

It is René Dubos' 1965 book, *Man Adapting*, that is continually cited as legitimizing and popularizing the image of the individual as a unit of adaptation—one in which health or disease are seen as a measure of the success or failure of an organism's efforts to respond to environmental challenges. Dubos was attempting to parallel Dobzhansky's (1962) work, *Mankind Evolving*, which dealt with the interplay between genetic endowment and environmental factors in humans, while, at the same time, shifting the focus from humankind as a whole to the individual human being: "*L'homme moyen sensuel*, trying as best he can to meet the emergencies of the day and to prepare for the uncertainties of the future" (p. xviii).

In the early 1960s, Dubos, already a renowned microbiologist for his work on antibiotics, was asked to give a series of presentations for the annual Sillman Foundation Lectures at Yale University, in conjunction with the 100th anniversary of the medical school. He used these lectures as a basis to broadly explore issues related to the interplay between humans and their environment while also addressing a growing concern of his with why bacteria, which at all times inhabit the human organism, only sometimes make people sick. This concern was based on his own research and on his wife's experience with tuberculosis during World War II, which Dubos described in a 1978 interview:

> Europe was at war. My first wife was French, born at Limoges. In 1939, at the beginning of the war, she came down with tuberculosis. I asked myself, "Why did she get tuberculosis, when we live as well as we do?" So I dug into her past and discovered that she'd had tuberculosis when she was about six or seven and had gotten well by herself, as most people do. Then why did she have a relapse? I theorized that the disasters in her family resulting from the war had caused her very great anguish. I'm convinced that this anguish reactivated the tuberculosis that to all appearances had been cured. She died three years later. (Piel & Segerberg, 1990, p. 10)

Over time, Dubos became more and more aware that:

> . . . prevalence and severity of microbial diseases were conditioned more by the ways of life of the persons afflicted than by the virulence and other properties of the etiological agents. Hence the need to learn more about man and his societies, in order to try to make sense of the patter of his diseases. (Dubos, 1965, p. xxi)

In *Man Adapting*, Dubos (1965) weaves together examples from an amazing cross-disciplinary base of historical, physiological, and social science research related to human adaptation at the population and individual levels. He examines evolutionary and nonevolutionary changes. In the process, he creates an image of humans as individuals who adapt to their environment in ways that create distinctive disease patterns across diverse environments. This is the process of adaptation.

Dubos (1965) saw the individual human being as responding to the total environment—physicochemical, biological, and social. Kim (1983) summarizes well the fullness of this image in this way:

> A person is thought to exercise adaptive abilities by selecting among alternatives to achieve a self-directed end, given the external conditions that are encountered at a given moment. Dubos' human, furthermore, is a product of the lasting and universal characteristics of human nature, inscribed in being, and yet is capable of establishing a personal history; thus, the person possesses both phylogenic and ontogenic adaptability. A person is seen as an organism responding to stimuli of environmental challenge in a manner that is based on rationality, i.e., that while some responses are based on the direct effects of the stimuli on the organism, most of a person's responses are usually determined not by such direct effects but by the symbolic interpretations he or she attaches to the stimuli.
>
> Thus, Dubos' human treats and responds to actual environmental stimuli in a chained sequence of direct reactions, indirect reactions that occur as ripple effects of the direct reactions, and responses to personalized symbols that are generated by the impinging stimuli. This human trait, according to Dubos, makes the individual's responses to any environmental factors extremely personal. (p. 49)

The major explanatory thrust of Dubos' (1965) argument begins with the environment. He gives extensive attention to the factors, especially physical and chemical properties in our air, water, and food, that directly and indirectly give rise to disease. His primary concern is on disease as the expression of the failure of the organism's efforts to respond adaptively to environmental challenges, although he acknowledges that survival and health are indicators of successful adaptation. In developing this argument, Dubos draws heavily on the physiological research and concepts of Cannon (1931) and Selye (1956) that contend that environment factors give rise to physiological stress in organisms and, in turn, make them more vulnerable to disease. Thus, an individual's perceptions and symbolic interpretations of their environments often are seen as playing a major role in an individual's response and, ultimately, are linked to the success or failure of that response.

For Dubos' (1965) intervention is aimed at helping "man function successfully in his environment—whether he is hunting the mammoth, toiling for his daily bread, or attempting to reach the moon" (p. xix).

ADAPTATION AND THEORY DEVELOPMENT IN NURSING

The most pervasive use of adaptation in the nursing literature is in the image it creates of the individual patient attempting to adjust to the peculiarities of a specific disease or disability. Dubos' (1965) depiction of the human being as continuously adapting to environmental challenges is embedded in this image. Disease is just one of the many that one must contend with in a lifetime. For most writers in nursing, human adaptation is more of an assumption, a belief, that undergirds educational curriculum and practice, than it is a scientific concept that can serve research and theory development.

However, for others, adaptation has presented a compelling theoretical framework to be used initially as a guide for integrating educational curricula and later for underpinning nursing research. In the early 1960s, as noted previously, adaptation was one of the first theoretical frameworks to be considered for undergirding nursing curricula. Much of this early writing included summaries of the existing theoretical and research literature on adaptation from outside nursing. Nursing scholars began pulling out the basic assumptions and major theoretical concepts and relationships that seemed to have particular relevance to nursing. At times, some authors went on to consider adaptation as a conceptual base for integrating other theoretical schools of though (e.g., socialization and individual psychodynamics).

In 1963, Pitel drew from the work of several well-established researchers, including Cannon (1932), Adolph (1956), and Selye (1956) to summarize the work being done on adaptation in physiology. She described the human being as a living organism adapting to an everchanging external environment via stimuli impinging on the organism and its internal environment. Adaptation was defined as the adjustment of the organism to environmental change. The focus was on identifying normal physiological regulatory and control mechanisms and then explaining how these enabled the organism to maintain a constant internal environment called homeostasis. Distinctions were made between environmental change of a short duration (such as daily fluctuations in outdoor temperatures), to those that persist for an "appreciable period of time" (e.g., high or low environmental temperatures of altitudes) and, lastly, to those that are of a "very severe nature" (i.e., the physical stress of intense heat or cold, trauma, restraint, or mental stress). It was in regard to the latter that Seyle's stress syndrome was seen as playing a role. According to Pitel:

> Any slight alteration of the internal environment (which may have originally arisen in the external environment) evokes regulatory responses to restore the internal environment to its original status. Cannon called this maintenance of a constant internal environment homeostasis. The adaptation is thus through internal regulation in the presence of environmental change. (Pitel, p. 263)

Pitel (1963) did not mention specific nursing interventions from this work. She simply suggested that nurses who possess this broad perspective, especially knowledge of normal regulatory and control mechanisms, would be better able to detect physiological deviations from the norm (such as partially developed, impaired, or completely lacking control mechanisms) and create more flexible care plans. Ideally these should take into account individual capabilities in adjusting to environmental change and helping individuals fit harmoniously with their environment. An example was given of the nurse who assists a patient in adjusting to life-supporting technology that was there to take the place of the patient's normal regulatory mechanisms.

In another article, Martin and Prange (1962) focused on the environmental changes that individuals normally encounter in their lives (i.e., birth, entering school, puberty, work and marriage, parenthood, involution, retirement, and death). They linked successful and unsuccessful attempts at adapting to these changes with states of health or illness, respectively. Others, for example, Vassallo (1965) and Levine (1966) were inspired by the publication of Dubos' (1965) *Man Adapting* as a basis for summarizing current thought on adaptation. Levine focused more on the underlying theoretical explanation in Dubos' work and applied this to patient responses to a cerebral vascular accident and how nursing care could be orchestrated across several phases of adaptation.

Still others began considering the possibility of integrating other existing theories within adaptation. Brown (1963) emphasized the "human organism's" capacity to learn and drew on theories of socialization from the writings of Talcott Parsons in sociology and George Herbert Mead in social psychology. She suggested that socialization could be seen as a major adaptive process that helps the individual become a social being and adapt to society by fulfilling roles and meeting the expectations of others, thereby maintaining integrity of personality. In a somewhat similar vein, but one driven more by psychiatry than sociology, Peplau (1963) focused on how individual behavior is molded over time and through an interpersonal field to gain a harmonious integration of behavior with that of others within the respective psychosocial field. From this angle, she suggested that "schizophrenia can be seen as massive ada chosocial behavior to overwhelmingly unfavorable conditio personal field" (p. 274). This constitutes an example of leading to the occurrence of a disease state. Peplau extrapola knowing the processes of adaptation underlying normal behav would be better able to understand the origins of the abnormal

A most systematic effort to develop a nursing theory with the conceptual focus on adaptation is seen in the Roy Adaptation Model. The Roy Adaptation Model proposed as a nursing framework by Callista Roy initially in 1970 and gone through some refinements (Roy, 1976; Roy, 1984; Roy & Andrews, 1991; Roy & Roberts, 1981) is basically based on the assumptions inherent in von Bertalanffy's general systems theory (1968) and Helson's adaptation level theory (1964). Roy views adaptation as a function of impinging stimuli and adaptation level which specifies where an individual is at a given moment in relation to all other preexisting stimuli and one's own internal resources. Hence, to Roy individuals are adaptive systems processing stimuli through coping mechanisms that are teleologically present in human beings. Human beings are adaptive in the sense that "the human system has the capacity to adjust effectively to changes in the environment and, in turn, affects the environment" (Roy & Andrews, 1991, p. 7). In combining the assumptions of the general systems theory and human adaptation, Roy proposes in her Roy Adaptation Model a view of human beings as systems receiving inputs as stimuli, processing them through the systems' internal and feedback mechanisms, and producing outputs as behaviors that can either be adaptive or ineffective. More specifically, she believes in the goal-directedness and teleological features of humans and views humans as systems processing "inputs," which are seen as a combined set of external stimuli and internal stimuli (equated as one's adaptation level at a given moment) through regulator and cognator mechanisms of coping.

Hence, to Roy the essence of human adaptation is in the interrelationships between the pooled effects of all stimuli of the environment (what she calls focal, contextual, and residual stimuli) and the individual's adaptation level, which is "the changing point that represents the person's ability to respond positively in a situation" (Roy & Andrews, 1991, p. 10). Behaviors as the outputs of coping are the responses of the adaptive system and reveal the nature of adapting by the human system to its environment. Behaviors as responses are either adaptive or ineffective in relation to whether they promote the person's integrity and the goals of adaptation. The human systems' goals of adaptation, according to Roy, are survival, growth, reproduction, and mastery. Therefore, to Roy adaptation

.efers to immediate, short-term responses to ever-changing environment, and "adaptive" has a positive connotation in relation to the system's preestablished goals. In elaborating the model, Roy added eight assumptions associated with humanism and veritivity to the basic tenets of the theory:

> In humanism, it is believed that the individual (a) shares in creative power, (b) behaves purposefully, not in a sequence of cause and effect, (c) possesses intrinsic holism, and (d) strives to maintain integrity and to realize the need for relationships. . . . In veritivity, it is believed that the individual in society is viewed in the context of the (a) purposefulness of human existence, (b) unity of purpose of humankind, (c) activity and creativity for the common good, and (d) value and meaning of life. (Roy & Andrews, 1991, p. 6)

Hence, entrenched within the coping mechanisms of regulator and cognator are the notions of creativity, communality of humans as social beings, and universal purpose of human kind. How such juxtapositioning influences the exact nature of adapting is unclear in the articulation of her model, however. In addition, how the universal goals of human systems and individual goals of adaptation play out in the process of adaptation for individuals in situations have not been specified in the Roy model. The picture emerging from the Roy Adaptation Model is a view of humans who exhibit behaviors that are either adaptive or ineffective judged by some external and objective criteria established in relation to the goals of adaptation. This makes the model to be circular in determining the nature of adaptation.

Other direct efforts besides that of Roy at using adaptation for theory development and research in nursing began in the 1980s. In contrast to Dubos' (1965) focus on processes giving rise to a disease, nurse theorists and researchers turned their attention to how individuals adapt to the disease condition itself. The general question has been how does any one individual adjust to a specific disease, disability, or medical treatment (e.g., an implantable cardioverter defibrillator) that represents some degree of permanent change? These are changes in which some time (anywhere from a few days to 2 years) is needed for the individual to reach the highest level of adjustment. Of these, the greatest attention by far has been on chronic or chronic-like disease (e.g., diabetes, epilepsy, or any one of many types of cancer).

Over the last 15 years, the more specific question has been why do some individuals do better than others? To address this question, nurses have identified a number of indicators and outcome measures to separate the successes from the failures in individuals' levels of adjustment. Measures have been used to cover physical or physiological adjustment (e.g., comorbidity indexes, activity scales, and lab values such as glycosylated hemoglobin levels for those with diabetes) and psychosocial adjustment (e.g., the psychosocial adjustment to illness scale and various measures of affect and depression) (Craney, 1997; Peterson, 1996; Wortel, 1995). A few have used a single measure, for example, Rosenberg's mastery scale or a quality of life questionnaire to capture an individual's overall adjustment (Crigger, 1993; Kessenich, 1997). Somewhat surprisingly, there has been very little debate in the literature about what it means to be *fit* or *adapted.*

A few scholars have focused on describing the overall process and identifying factors that influence it, for example, Reed (1997) and Dwyer (1993) on one aspect of the adaptation process (i.e., Wiklinski's phenomenological study of the use of humor among patients with cancer). Most, however, have looked at the process from a quantitative and explanatory angle. Some have drawn on loose theoretical notions from Dubos' (1965) work, for example, Warner (1996), Peterson (1996), and Wortel (1995), while most have used specific theories of coping and adaptation (e.g., Lazarus & Folkman's theory of stress and coping, Taylor's theory of cognitive adaptation, Roy's adaptation theory) on which to build their hypotheses. When using one of the coping theories, researchers usually use the term *adaptation* to refer to the outcome and *coping* to refer to the process.

The role of the environment is not easy to decipher in the above research, although it is clear that the classic way of looking at environment and adaptation, as influencing disease patterns, is of very low, if any, interest to nursing scholars. Environment is rarely identified as a central concept in explaining why some adjust better than others. Instead, variables, such as social support, are considered to be potential resources within the environment that act as facilitators in patients' efforts to adjust rather than the major element to which the patient is adjusting.

REFERENCES

Adolph, E. F. (1956). General and specific characteristics of physiological adaptations. *American Journal of Physiology, 184,* 18–28.

Alland, A., Jr., & McCay, B. (1973). The concept of adaptation in biological and cultural evolution. In J. J. Honigmann (Ed.), *Handbook of social and cultural anthropology* (pp. 143–178). Chicago: Rand McNally.

Brown, M. I. (1963, October–November). Socialization—A social theory of adaptation. *Nursing Science,* pp. 280–294.

Cannon, W. B. (1931). *The wisdom of the body.* New York: Norton.

Cannon, W. B. (1932). *The wisdom of the body.* New York: Norton.

Carneiro, R. L. (1973). The four faces of evolution. In J. J. Honigmann (Ed.), *Handbook of social and cultural anthropology* (pp. 89–110). Chicago: Rand McNally.

Craney, J. M. (1997). Implantable cardioverter defibrillators and their physical and psychosocial outcomes. (Doctoral Dissertation, Boston College, 1996). *Dissertation Abstracts B, 57*(10), 6175.

Crigger, N. J. (1993). An adaptation model for women with multiple sclerosis. (Doctoral Dissertation, University of Florida, 1992). *Dissertation Abstracts B, 54*(5), 2437.

Darwin, C. (1859). *The origin of species by means of natural selection or the preservation of favored races in the struggle for life.* London: J. Murray.

Dobzhansky, T. (1962). *Mankind evolving.* New Haven, CT: Yale University Press.

Dubos, R. (1965). *Man adapting.* New Haven, CT: Yale University Press.

Dwyer, M. L. (1993). The oncology patient's experiences in making a treatment decision. (Doctoral Dissertation, The Catholic University of America, 1993). *Dissertation Abstracts B, 54*(3), 1330.

Eisenstadt, S. N. (1968). Social evolution. In *International encyclopedia of the social sciences* (Vol. 3, pp. 228–234). New York: Macmillan and Free Press.

Encyclopedia of sociology. (1974). Guilford, CT: Dushkin.

Hall, B. A. (1991). Adaptability: A personal resource of health. *Scholarly Inquiry in Nursing Practice, 5*(2), 95–112.

Harris, M. (1968). *The rise of anthropological theory: A history of theories of culture.* New York: Crowell.

Helson, H. H. (1964). *Adaptation level theory.* New York: Harper & Row.

Kessenich, C. R. (1997). Quality of life of elderly women with spinal fractures secondary to osteoporosis. (Doctoral Dissertation, University of Alabama at Birmingham, 1996). *Dissertation Abstracts B, 57*(8), 4976.

Kim, H. S. (1983). *The nature of theoretical thinking in nursing.* Norwalk, CT: Appleton-Century-Crofts.

Lenski, G., Lenski, J., & Nolan, P. (1995). *Human societies: An introduction to macrosociology* (7th ed.). New York: McGraw-Hill.

Lerner, M. L. (1968). *Heredity, evolution and society.* San Francisco: Freeman.

Levine, M. E. (1966). Adaptation and assessment: A rationale for nursing intervention. *American Journal of Nursing, 66*, 2450–2453.

Martin, H. W., & Prange, A. J., Jr. (1962). Human adaptation: A conceptual approach to understanding patients. *The Canadian Nurse, 58*, 243–243.

McElroy, A., & Townsend, P. K. (1996). *Medical anthropology in ecological perspective.* Boulder, CO: Westview.

Parsons, T. (1964). Evolutionary universals in society. *American Sociological Review, 29,* 339–357.

Peplau, H. E. (1963). Interpersonal relations and the process of adaptation. *Nursing Science, 1,* 272–279.

Peterson, J. Z. (1996). Changes in hope and coping in older adults during rehabilitation after hip fracture. (Doctoral Dissertation, University of Florida, 1995). *Dissertation Abstracts B, 57*(2), 991.

Piel, G., & Segerberg, O., Jr. (1990). *The world of Rene Dubos: A collection from his writings.* New York: Henry Holt and Company.

Pitel, M. (1963, October–November). Physiological adaptation in man. *Nursing Science,* pp. 263–271.

Reed, D. B. (1997). Occupational rehabilitation of farmers with upper-extremity amputations. (Doctoral Dissertation, University of Kentucky, 1996). *Dissertation Abstracts B, 57*(9), 5577.

Roy, C. (1976). *Introduction to nursing: An adaptation model.* Englewood Cliffs, NJ: Prentice-Hall.

Roy, C. (1984). *Introduction to nursing: An adaptation model.* 2nd ed. Englewood Cliffs, NJ: Prentice-Hall.

Roy, C., & Andrews, H. A. (1991). *The Roy adaptation model: The definitive statement.* Norwalk, CT: Appleton & Lange.

Roy, C., & Roberts, S. L. (1981). *Theory construction in nursing: An adaptation model.* Englewood Cliffs, NJ: Prentice-Hall.

Selye, H. O. (1956). *The stress of life.* New York: McGraw-Hill.

Service, E. R. (1968). Cultural evolution. In *International encyclopedia of the social sciences* (Vol. 3, pp. 221–227). New York: Macmillan and Free Press.

Vassallo, C. (1965, August). A concept of health. *Nursing Science,* pp. 236–242.

von Bertalanffy, L. (1968). *General system theory: Foundations, development, applications.* New York: Braziller.

Warner, L. S. (1996). The relationship of selected psychosocial and pathophysiological variables to depression in epilepsy patients. (Doctoral Dissertation, The Catholic University of America, 1996). *Dissertation Abstracts B, 57*(5), 3132.

Washburn, S. L., & Lancaster, J. B. (1968). Human evolution. In *International encyclopedia of the social sciences* (Vol. 3, pp. 215–221). New York: Macmillan and Free Press.

Wortel, L. H. (1995). The physiological and psychosocial adaptation of individuals with insulin-dependent diabetes and non-insulin dependent diabetes. (Doctoral Dissertation, University of Miami, 1994). *Dissertation Abstracts B, 55*(7), 2651.

3

Human Needs and Nursing Theory

Jacqueline Fortin

The concept of *human needs*, as it relates to nursing practice and theory construction, does not lend itself to clear and unambiguous definition. Rather, the literature reveals two major and often competing facets: that of a motivational drive that directs human behavior and that of a force—politically driven and socially and culturally shaped. The two facets, however, are not necessarily independent. Holmes and Warelow (1997) have, in fact, described them as reflexive. It is viewed to be reflexive because human needs defined as desires or wants shape the emergence of political and social policies. In turn, political ideologies and social and cultural forces shape the perceived needs of individuals or groups. Both facets, alone or considered together, play an important role in the conceptualization of needs as it relates to current nursing practice and nursing theory development.

From a scientific stance, the concept of human needs is of necessity an invented abstraction ultimately defined within the parameters of the scientists' disciplinary alliance (e.g., biology, psychology, sociology, anthropology, nursing, or political science), theoretical orientation, and world view. The concerns of those in the biological sciences evolve around physiological or somatic needs related to survival and health. Psychologists tend to expand the repertoire of needs to include higher level needs, such as esteem; while social scientists place these and other social needs (e.g., affiliation) into the context of social interaction, culture, or international politics. While each of these perspectives is to varying degrees important to nursing practice and theory development, traditionally, nurse theorists have tended to draw mainly from needs theories that reflect objective, individualist accounts such as those of Abraham Maslow. Only recently has nursing begun to take note of the importance of social and political forces within health care in general and nursing in particular (see for example, Holmes & Warelow, 1997; Yura & Walsh, 1988).

The broader conceptualization provides opportunity for exploring "images and details that are not readily apparent when viewed from one perspective" (Meleis, 1991, p. 249). For example, the broader conceptualization suggests a need for historical review and the need to distinguish human needs from socially constructed wants, desires, and satisfiers. At the same time, it raises cogent questions regarding the universality of needs, their contextual dependence, and their distinctly Western bias.

These issues are discussed in the first section of this chapter. Questions are raised rather than answered. The second section of the chapter presents an overview of nursing's needs theories with attention to how they are evolving.

CONCEPTUALIZATIONS OF HUMAN NEEDS

Marx (1964) was among the first modern theorists to link human needs to social and political forces. He proposed that the ideal society was one that recognized the needs of the people and fulfilled them. In contrast, Sites (1992) notes that Parsons and other sociologists took the position that biogenetic needs are transformed into need dispositions through the socialization process. Thus, "all explanation can be reduced to the social or cultural order under the assumption that humans are infinitely malleable" (p. 179). Malinowski attempted to define human nature by listing basic needs at various systems levels. He maintained that biological health was a necessity if social structural integrity and cultural unity were to be met (Turner, 1991b).

Since Marx and Malinowski, a host of scholars have attempted to tie social, cultural, and political forces to what is often characterized as the innate nature of man (Montagu, 1955) reflected either as a single human need—for adequacy (Combs, Richards, & Richards, 1976)—or as a list of multiple needs that address those of the individual, family, community, and the nation (see for example, McHale & McHale, 1978).

The mid to late 1970s saw an increased interest in human needs as they relate to the allocation of services and resources in both developed and developing nations. As human needs theories began to take on international significance, the tendency to reflect a Western bias became increasingly apparent (for a comprehensive discussion of this topic, see Galtung, 1980). As one example, Lederer (1980b), based on personal communication with Dr. Kinhide Mushakoji, notes that the Japanese language has no word comparable to need. "(W)henever one tries to translate 'needs' into Japanese, something like wants, wishes, or desires will come out" (p. 8) making communication of needs difficult if not impossible. One can assume that this would be problematic in other cultures as well. Analyzing Westernization from a different perspective, Holmes and Warelow (1997) chide Yura and Walsh for their "thinly disguised middle class liberal American ideology" (p. 461) in the development of their eclectic theory of human needs. Here, the problem is not communication but, rather, the conceptualization of how needs are satisfied. Specifically, Yura and Walsh (1988) characterize the family as the "primary unit for human need fulfillment" (p. 96) although they recognize the role of the community, state, nation, and so on in facilitating need fulfillment.

Critics of Westernization challenge the underlying premise of the universality of basic human needs. They contend that such lists imply a model to be imitated by other cultures. Other questions revolve around the analytic stance toward epistemology that Westerners take. A list of needs and categories of needs can only be conceptualized as components or dimensions of a whole. Such conceptualizations can be problematic for scientists attempting to describe the holistic experiences (Galtung, 1980). As Galtung notes, however, the

> analytic versus holistic image is not a dichotomy of alternatives; it . . . can be seen as a both-and rather than an either-or. . . . The problem is not how to suppress analytic thinking in this field, but how to facilitate and promote holistic thinking. (p. 82)

Despite concerns of Western bias, most scholars agree that all humans possess certain organic or "basic needs" that must be satisfied for the sake of physical health (Mallmann & Marcus, 1980) and survival (Lederer, 1980a; Malinowski, 1944; Maslow, 1968, 1970; Montagu, 1955). However, McHale and McHale (1978) and others argue that people have desires and aspirations that go beyond physiologic or somatic needs and that the consequences, when these needs are not met, may be equally dire. Needs for social interaction, for example, are necessary for psychological well being (Turner, 1987, 1991a, 1991b) and when not met may lead to feelings of loneliness and isolation (Linton, 1945), therefore, threatening mental health. Less clear, perhaps, is the proposed interplay between the organic needs of individuals and their related satisfiers.

Personal, cultural, and societal values have a substantial influence on what is defined as a need and what mechanisms are considered appropriate for its satisfaction (McHale & McHale, 1978; Yura & Walsh, 1988).

Montagu (1955) points out that while culture may play no role in the innate structure of a need, "(n)eeds function in a culture and culture modifies them" (p. 135). Others argue that it is not needs that are modified by social forces but their expressions as wants, wishes, desires, aspirations, and satisfiers. This stance begs the question as to whether it is possible to distinguish needs from these related concepts.

ARE NEEDS OBJECTIVE AND UNIVERSAL?

The question of whether human needs are universal and objective is a poignant one and one that has engendered much scholarly debate. Some authors (see for example, McHale & McHale, 1978; Montagu, 1955, 1966) suggest that individual needs vary enormously in kind and in quality and particularly in relationship to the life cycle. But Linton (1945) and others (e.g., Watt, 1996) would argue that it is not the need that varies but rather the behaviors that the need gives rise to. Thus, authors who favor the universal and objective conceptualization of needs contend that it is not the notion of needs that is subjective, but rather the related desires and satisfiers—that according to Lederer (1980b) "differ in terms of space, time, and culture" (p. 5). It is the incorrect use of the term need, Mallmann and Marcus (1980) suggest, that is the basis for the terminological and conceptual confusion so prevalent in needs research.

Lederer (1980a) draws on the terminology used by Mallmann and Marcus (1980) who espouse to a universal and objective notion of needs. These authors characterize needs as "universal; and desires and satisfiers as spatially, temporally, and personally" determined (p. 166). They contend that "There is no one-to-one relation between needs and desires. Many desires are just distortions of needs" (p. 167). Mallmann and Marcus further maintain that individual attitudes are expressed by desires, whereas, needs are an expression of universal human requirements—requirements of which people may not be aware. Therefore, it is desires and satisfiers that theorists of the historical/subjective school are striving to understand and explain. For it is desires and satisfiers that are socially constructed and without objective content. The latter are linked with subjective feelings, and whereas individuals may not be conscious of their needs, they can readily articulate their correlated wants, desires, and satisfiers (Galtung, 1980). If we accept the distinction between needs and desires (satisfiers), we have a sound basis for the integration of the two needs approaches, the "universal/objective" and the "historical/subjective" (Lederer, 1980b, p. 8).

Holmes and Warelow (1997) take a different view. These authors suggest that if we accept the notion of reflexive interplay between needs and social context the search for universal need is futile. And that would surely be the case if we accepted the premise, put forth by Plant and colleagues, that needs are socially constructed and cannot be readily differentiated from wants (Plant, Lesser, & Taylor-Gooby as cited in Holmes & Warelow, 1980). It could be argued, however, that if we accept that the reflexive interplay is not between need and social context, but rather, between the two facets of human need—one a motivational drive and the other a socially shaped force—then we could view them as two sides to one coin. From this perspective, desires, wants, and satisfiers would be viewed as variables subject to manipulation. Motivational drives would be considered universal and designated as human needs. This does not mean that a comprehensive list of all basic human needs is possible or even desirable, "but it does make sense to talk about certain classes of needs, such as, 'security needs,' . . . 'identity meeds,' " (Galtung, 1980, p. 59) that will be experienced at some time by human beings everywhere, and to differentiate these from desires and satisfiers. Katrin Lederer (1980b) provides the following example:

> "I need a car," according to the above understanding would not be a needs statement. The person desires a car. The car is a satisfier. What the person might need is, for example, mobility, or status, or (speed-)ecstasy. Under the person's personal set of living conditions, a car might be the adequate satisfier to meet any of the needs mentioned. (p. 5)

IS THERE A HIERARCHY OF NEEDS?

The most pervasive assumption, whether implicit or explicit, in theories of human need is that of a needs hierarchy. The physiological needs linked to survival of the individual or group are usually addressed first with the connotation that they should be satisfied first, prior to higher level mental or spiritual needs (Galtung, 1980; Maslow, 1970). For example, Montagu (1955, 1966) draws on the work of Malinowski to propose a two-structure hierarchy. The first level reflects "vital" basic human needs (e.g., for sleep, ingestion of food, activity, and escape from danger). These basic needs, Montagu (1966) maintains, constitute the minimum biological conditions that must be satisfied by any living group if its members are to survive. The second level of the hierarchy addresses "non vital" basic human needs, such as those related to security and social recognition, which must be satisfied if the individual "is to develop and maintain adequate mental health."

In a somewhat similar fashion, McHale and McHale (1978) propose that "sufficiency" and "growth" needs constitute a "second floor" in the needs hierarchy. Unlike basic universal needs, these second floor needs are defined by each society for its members.

There is also a clear hierarchy in the human need system offered by Carlos Mallmann (1980), who classifies human needs according to four categories. Needs that are necessary for (a) existence (subsistence and security), (b) coexistence (belongingness and esteem), (c) growth (development and renewal), and (d) perfection (transcendence and maturity). Mallmann contends that satisfaction of each of the eight needs is a requirement if one is to avoid illness. Galtung (1980) also produced a hierarchical list of basic human needs that he placed into four categories: security, welfare, identity, and freedom. Specific needs within each category bring the list to 28. Perhaps the author most often associated with a hierarchical structure of needs is Abraham Maslow.

Maslow

Unlike the social and political science scholars noted above, Maslow (1968, 1970) provides a set of objective "basic human needs" that reflect a different discipline, theoretical orientation, and world view. For example, Maslow's (1954) seminal work on motivation and personality provided the contextual underpinnings from which his hierarchical model of human needs evolved. Educated as a psychologist, Maslow depicted the basic human needs as those necessary for survival or those needs that would produce frustration or psychopathology if not met.

Consistent with his interest in psychopathology, Maslow (1954) put aside, as many other clinical psychologists have done, the less understood cognitive and aesthetic needs, designating them as "prerequisites for the basic need satisfactions" (p. 92). Therefore, the cognitive desires to know and to understand and the overlapping aesthetic needs become part of the "gestalt" in Maslow's holistic dynamic view of personality.

Maslow's (1954, 1968, 1970) scientific philosophy or world view emanates from organismic theory. His conception of man is that of a "whole, functioning, adjusting individual" (1954, p. 25) who can best be understood from a holistic-analytic style. One essential characteristic of this form of analysis is its dependence on understanding the whole. However, to understand the dynamic whole one must understand the role that any given part plays within the gestalt of the whole. That is, the whole and its parts are mutually related; the whole is necessary to an understanding of the part, and, in turn, the parts are necessary to an understanding of the whole. Based on organismic theory, Maslow proposed five basic human needs: physiological needs, safety needs, belongingness and love needs, esteem needs, and needs for self-actualization. According to Maslow, these needs constitute an inexact hierarchy beginning with the physiological needs and culminating in a drive for self-actualization.

Consistent with the physiological needs described by the authors cited above, Maslow's list includes the somatically based drives of hunger, thirst, sexual desire, and the need for rest, sleep, exercise and so on. Gratification of these physiological needs paves the way for satisfaction of the more socially oriented needs for safety and security. As physiological and safety needs are met, at least to some degree, needs for belongingness and love, self-esteem, and the desire for self-actualization emerge (Maslow, 1970). Leidy (1994) brings our attention to the fact that "(a)lthough Maslow's theory is frequently cited in the nursing literature and is commonly used as an underlying framework for clinical practice, it has been subjected to limited empirical scrutiny" (p. 277). This criticism has been echoed by Holmes and Warelow (1997) and Minshull, Ross, and Turner (1986) as well.

While there appears to be general agreement among the authors reviewed here, it is important to note that currently there is no scientific basis for establishing a hierarchy of importance, particularly in higher level needs. While intuitively most authors would agree that it is more pressing for organic needs and safety needs to be met than higher level needs, they do not maintain that people pursue maximum satisfaction of all of their organic needs before giving attention to those needs often characterized as higher level. Further, the expression of human needs (wants, desires, satisfiers) and the gestalt of their interdependence will vary between individuals and groups over time and under varying conditions.

For example, McHale and McHale (1978) address the dimensions of international poverty and the dire social consequences when basic human needs go unmet. Taking into account the interdependence of needs, these authors reflect on the vicious cycle that occurs in situations of social and economic deprivation. In relation to health, they note that: "Poor nutrition lowers disease resistance. Hunger and ill-health impair productivity which, in turn, lessens the capacity to secure more food . . . and be more resistant to disease" (p. 31).

HUMAN NEEDS THEORIES IN NURSING

In 1991, Meleis carried out a comprehensive analysis of nursing theories developed between 1950 and 1970. When their paradigmatic origins, time and period of development, central questions, and central concepts, were taken into consideration, three distinct schools of thought emerged: needs, interaction, and outcome. The school of thought associated with needs "developed in response to the question 'What do nurses do?' " (p. 251). Thus, Meleis identifies Henderson, Abdellah, and Orem as "needs theorists": Henderson's position emphasizes the nurses' role in complementing and supplementing individual's needs to maintain independence, while Abdellah specifies human's need-related problems as the focus of nursing attention, and Orem conceptualizes her theory around the concept of self-care needs (1991, pp. 252–254). Theorists, within this school, namely Henderson, Abdellah, and Orem, described the potential functions and roles of nurses in terms of patient needs, loosely based "on the fundamental needs of man" (Thorndike as cited in Henderson, 1991, p. 16) or Maslow's hierarchy. Thus, needs theorists provided us with a "view of human beings that was slightly different but very close to the view provided by the biomedical model" (Meleis, 1991, p. 252).

The pioneering efforts of these theorists provide an excellent example of the reflexive nature of needs. Namely, it reflects the interplay between the two facets of needs discussed above: one that is viewed as an internal motivational drive and another that is viewed as politically driven and socially and culturally shaped. In particular, the latter is clearly demonstrated in the works of Henderson (1991) and Abdellah (Abdellah & Levine, 1986). The needs theories developed by these two theorists were, in part, shaped by the social and political forces that had come to bear on the profession as a result of "technological advancement and social change" (Dycus, Schmeiser, & Yancy, 1986, p. 94).

One driving social force undergirding the development of Henderson's and Abdellah's models was the recognition by the profession that changes in professional status could only be brought about by defining a scientific body of knowledge, a body of knowledge unique to nursing. A key objective, therefore, of these early efforts was to formulate models that were patient centered and that promoted independent nursing practice. The notion of need as a motivational drive that directs human behavior and that elicits consequences when the need is unmet provided a potential seedbed for such a model. Based on a conceptualization of the client in terms of human needs and the nurse as one who could provide care when needs were unmet, these efforts were translated into Henderson's (1991)

14 conditions and Abdellah's (Abdellah, Beland, Martin, & Matheny, 1960) typology of 21 nursing problems. The ultimate goal was to bring about radical change in nursing education and nursing practice.

Although Abdellah's writings are not specific as to theoretical statements, thoughtful analysis and critique of her works (e.g., Abdellah, 1957; Abdellah, Beland, Martin, & Metheny, 1960; Abdellah & Levine, 1986) by several nurse scholars (see for example, Dycus, Schmeiser, & Yancy, 1986; Falco, 1995; Meleis, 1991; See, 1989) help to provide the context within which her typology of 21 problems was developed.

In response to the demand for problem-centered approaches in nursing education and nursing practice, Abdellah set out to develop a model that reflected scientific knowledge unique to nursing. She conducted descriptive investigations designed to explicate health care situations that are problematic to the patient or family and that are amenable to the professional functions of the nurse (See, 1989). The concepts, grounded in empirical data, formed categories that reflected needs, deficits, and problems that, in turn, provided the structure for the empirical listing of 21 groups of common nursing problems. Consistent with Maslow's (1954) theoretical orientation, the client is viewed as a whole made up of physiological, sociological, and psychological parts. This conceptualization of the client, along with types of interpersonal relationships between the nurse and patient, and common elements of patient care laid the groundwork for Abdellah's typology of 21 nursing problems listed below (Abdellah, Beland, Martin, & Matheny, 1960):

1. To maintain good hygiene and physical comfort.
2. To promote optimal activity; exercise, rest, and sleep.
3. To promote safety through prevention of accident, injury, or other trauma and through the prevention of the spread of infection.
4. To maintain good body mechanics and prevent and correct deformities.
5. To facilitate the maintenance of a supply of oxygen to all body cells.
6. To facilitate the maintenance of nutrition of all body cells.
7. To facilitate the maintenance of elimination.
8. To facilitate the maintenance of fluid and electrolyte balance.
9. To recognize the physiological responses of the body to disease conditions—pathological, physiological, and compensatory.
10. To facilitate the maintenance of regulatory mechanisms and functions.
11. To facilitate the maintenance of sensory function.

12. To identify and accept positive and negative expressions, feelings, and reactions.
13. To identify and accept the interrelatedness of emotions and organic illness.
14. To facilitate the maintenance of effective verbal and nonverbal communication.
15. To promote the development of productive interpersonal relationships.
16. To facilitate progress toward achievements of personal spiritual goals.
17. To create and/or maintain a therapeutic environment.
18. To facilitate awareness of self as an individual with varying physical, emotional, and developmental needs.
19. To accept the optimum possible goals in the light of limitations, physical and emotional.
20. To use community resources as an aid in resolving problems arising from illness.
21. To understand the role of social problems as influencing factors in the cause of illness (pp. 126–127).

Abdellah and Levine (1986) offer the list of 21 problems without defining the relationship of needs to problems. She does, however, characterize them as an "overt" or "covert" nursing problem or "a condition faced by the patient or family which the nurse can assist him or them to meet through the performance of her professional functions" (p. 54).

There is general agreement among nurse scholars that health, nursing problem, and problem solving are the three major concepts in Abdellah's writings (see for example, Dycus, Schmeiser, & Yancy, 1986; Falco, 1995; Meleis, 1991; See, 1989). Health is loosely defined by Abdellah as a reflection of "(s)elf-help ability developed and maintained at a level at which need satisfaction can take place without assistance" (Abdellah & Levine, 1986, p. 54). In earlier writings, Abdellah and colleagues (1960) linked health to need satisfaction; she did not, however, as See (1989) notes "explicate in detail the distinction between satisfying health needs and nursing problems" (p. 128). While there is no explicit mention of a hierarchy of needs, Abdellah indicated that "when for some reason any of these necessities—air, water, food, temperature, intactness of body tissue—departs from the optimum, a state of need can be said to exist" (Abdellah, Beland, Martin, & Matheney, 1960, p. 53). This would suggest that she considered some needs as vital needs in contrast to those considered less vital, such as esteem needs.

The conceptualization of nursing problems is less clear and has generated dialogue as to the primary thrust of the model. Abdellah and Levine (1986) define nursing problem as "a condition faced by the patient or family which the nurse can assist him or them to meet through performance of professional functions" (p. 54). Falco (1995) argues that, contrary to the client-centered orientation that Abdellah professes to, this definition "is more consistent with 'nursing functions' or 'nursing goals' than with client-centered problems" (p. 145). Consequently, the more nursing-centered orientation tends to magnify the concept of problem solving and the role of the nurse in the health care relationship. So, despite her stated shift from nursing problems to patient-client condition and outcomes (Abdellah & Levine, 1986), "scrutiny of the problem solving concept somewhat obscures the original intent of the model which was apparently to emphasize . . . the special patient condition which responds to nursing intervention" (See, 1989, p. 130). From this latter perspective the clients' condition would be viewed as problems (needs) that act as a cue to guide nursing assessment and interventions.

Problem solving provides the final building block to Abdellah's writing. Defined as the process of identifying overt and covert problems, it is based on the assumption that correct identification of nursing problems, which may be emotional, sociological, or interpersonal in nature, is crucial to selecting the appropriate course of action (Falco, 1995).

Abdellah's model, in particular her list of 21 problems, is generally characterized as one based on Maslow's hierarchy of needs. While the relationship between the conceptualizations of the two authors is sketchy, to her credit there is not an over emphasis on lower level needs. In fact, many fall into the category of esteem needs and belonging and love (affiliation) needs.

There are notable similarities between Abdellah's 21 problems and Henderson's (1991) 14 components of basic nursing care. There are also, however, distinct differences. Henderson's components are clearly client centered and considered in the context of four factors always present: (a) age; (b) temperament, emotional state, or passing mood; (c) social or cultural status; and (d) physical and intellectual capacity. In contrast, Abdellahs problems tend to be more nurse-centered, focused on nursing problems and nursing service. Henderson's 14 components of nursing care reflect her view of humans as biological, psychological, sociological, and spiritual beings. The basic needs of humans are reflected in the 14 components. However, congruent with the needs theorists, she notes that "these needs are satisfied by infinitely varied patterns of living, no two of which are alike" (Henderson, 1991, p. 3).

Henderson views health in the context of human functioning. According to Furukawa and Howe (1995), "(h)er definition of health is based on the individual's ability to function independently, as outlined in the 14 components" (p. 74). When the individual is unable to perform those activities independently it is the nurse's duty to assist that individual (Henderson, 1991). To carry out this function, "(f)or Henderson the nurse must be knowledgeable, have some base for practicing individualized and humane care, and be a scientific problem solver" (Furukawa & Howe, 1995, p. 75).

The concept of needs is neither defined nor discussed in any depth by either Henderson or Abdellah. However, it is important to remember that their focus was not on psychological theories of human behavior, but rather client problems, nursing education, and nursing practice. Nonetheless, assumptions about the nature of humans and their needs influence implicitly and perhaps without awareness, our theoretical thinking. Abraham Maslow (as cited in Wrightsman, 1992) wrote:

> Every psychologist, however positivistic and antitheoretical he may claim to be has a full blown philosophy of human nature hidden away within him. It is as if he guided himself by a half-known map, which he disavows and denies, and which is therefore immune to intrusion or correction by newly acquired knowledge. (p. 38)

In any event, Abdellah and Henderson had a significant impact on nursing education and nursing practice. Their successes laid the groundwork for future generations.

CURRENT CONTEXTUAL FEATURES

The 1970s to the 1990s saw a number of relevant changes in nursing and the conceptualization of human needs. Nursing's earlier goals for defining a unique body of knowledge to guide practice and education had come to fruition and has become increasingly institutionalized in the nursing process. Scholarly debate has turned to issues of philosophy, research methodology, holism, interpretivism, and so on. At the same time, theories addressing human needs were maturing. The initial focus on the individual and innate motivational drives broadened to include the political and social issues that the notion of basic human needs raises. The debate has moved to issues such as universality, with some authors arguing that human needs are not universal, objective, or innate, but socially, culturally, and politically derived. Thus concerns about delivery of care have given way to those addressing access to care. While the jury is still out on this issue, and questions regarding the hierarchy of needs, interdependence of needs, importance of contextual features, and the term differentiated from wants, desires, or satisfiers are emerging.

The work of Yura and Walsh (1978, 1988) draws on the broader conceptualization of human needs theory and recognizes its influence on nursing process. Suggesting that "the integrity of all of the human needs of the person(s) is the territory of nursing" (p. 70), these authors proposed an eclectic theory of human needs. Drawing on a number of international need theorists (e.g., Galtung, Mallmann, Maslow, McHale & McHale, Montagu) for theoretical substance, Yura and Walsh identified 35 human needs of the client (person, family, and community). Unlike the Abdellah and Henderson theories, Yura and Walsh (1988) define need. Paraphrasing Montagu (1955) they note that:

> Proponents of human need theory view the person as an integrated, organized whole who is motivated toward meeting human needs. A human need is viewed as an internal tension that results in an alteration in some state of the system. This tension expresses itself in goal-directed behavior. (Yura & Walsh, 1988, p. 70)

Working from this basic definition these authors define their 35 problems in the context of the social and cultural insights wrought from their comprehensive literature review.

From a different perspective, Holmes and Warelow (1997) state that "needs . . . are always socially constructed" (p. 469). Therefore, they recommend making critical theory a force for change. They note that there are two key tasks that critical theory must undertake: "first, the formulation of a theory of the good life and its relation to needs, commodities and consumption and, second, the clarification of the relationship between theory and practice" (p. 467). In addition, they recommend "praxis," a concept well known to nurses, as a method for "restructuring need interpretations" (p. 468).

The philosophical and theoretical differences between Holmes and Warelow (1997) and Yura and Walsh (1988) are provocative and highlight the two distinctly different approaches to human needs conceptualizations that are emerging. For Yura and Walsh needs reside within the individual and those needs when unmet guide practice. In contrast, Holmes and Warelow view human needs as potent political and ethical issues that are socially constructed. No doubt more nurse scholars will enter the arena of needs theorizing as issues of access to care, treatment options, advanced technology, assisted suicide, and starvation move to the forefront of health care and nursing in the next millennium. That, however, does not negate our need to continue to explore avenues to understanding the human needs of our clients (individuals, family, community) and how those needs can best be met, for that is not only the unique function of nursing, it is nursing's social mandate.

REFERENCES

Abdellah, F. G. (1957). Methods of identifying covert aspects of nursing problems: A key to improved clinical teaching. *Nursing Research, 6*(11), 4–23.

Abdellah, F. G., Beland, I. L., Martin, A., & Metheney, R. V. (1960). *Patient centered approaches to nursing*. New York: Macmillan.

Abdellah, F. G., & Levine, E. (1986). *Better patient care through nursing research* (3rd ed.). New York: Macmillan.

Combs, A. W., Richards, A. C., & Richards, F. (1976). *Perceptual psychology: A humanistic approach to the study of persons.* New York: Harper & Row.

Dycus, D. K., Schmeiser, D. N., & Yancy, R. (1986). Faye Glenn Abdellah. In A. Marriner (Ed.), *Nursing theorists and their work* (pp. 93–101). St. Louis, MO: Mosby.

Falco, S. M. (1995). Faye Glenn Abdellah. In J. B. George (Ed.), *Nursing theories: The base for professional nursing practice* (4th ed., pp. 143–158). Norwalk, CT: Appleton & Lange.

Furukawa, C. Y., & Howe, J. K. (1995). Virginia Henderson. In J. B. George (Ed.), *Nursing theories: The base for professional nursing practice* (4th ed., pp. 67–85). Norwalk, CT: Appleton & Lange.

Galtung, J. (1980). The basic needs approach. In K. Lederer (Ed.), *Human needs: A contribution to the current debate* (pp. 55–130). Cambridge, UK: Oelgeschlager, Gunn & Hain.

Henderson, V. A. (1991). *The nature of nursing: Reflections after 25 years.* New York: National League of Nursing Press.

Holmes, C. A., & Warelow, P. J. (1997). Culture, needs and nursing: A critical theory approach. *Journal of Advanced Nursing, 25,* 463–470.

Lederer, K. (Ed.). (1980a). *Human needs: A contribution to the current debate.* In K. Lederer (Ed.), *Human needs: A contribution to the current debate* (pp. 1–18). Cambridge, UK: Oelgeschlager, Gunn & Hain.

Lederer, K. (1980b). Needs methodology: The environmental case. In K. Lederer (Ed.), *Human needs: A contribution to the current debate* (pp. 259–278). Cambridge, UK: Oelgeschlager, Gunn & Hain.

Leidy, N. K. (1994). Operationalizing Maslow's theory: Developing and testing of the Basic Need Satisfaction Inventory. *Issues in Mental Health Nursing, 15,* 277–295.

Linton, R. (1945). *The cultural background of personality.* New York: Appleton-Century-Crofts.

Malinowski, B. (1944). *A scientific theory of culture and other essays.* Chapel Hill, NC: University of North Carolina Press.

Mallmann, C. A. (1980). Society, needs, and rights: A systematic approach. In K. Lederer (Ed.)., *Human needs: A contribution to the current debate* (pp. 37–54). Cambridge, UK: Oelgeschlager, Gunn & Hain.

Mallmann, C. A., & Marcus, S. (1980). Logical clarifications in the study of needs. In K. Lederer (Ed.)., *Human needs: A contribution to the current debate* (pp. 163–185). Cambridge, UK: Oelgeschlager, Gunn & Hain.

Marx, K. (1964). *Economic and philosophical manuscripts of 1844* (M. Milligam, Trans.). New York: International Publishers. (Original work published 1844).

Maslow, A. (1968). *Toward a psychology of being.* New York: Van Nostrand Reinhold.

Maslow, A. (1970). *Motivation and personality* (2nd ed.). New York: Harper & Row.

Maslow, A. H. (1954). *Motivation and personality.* New York: Harper & Brothers.

McHale, J., & McHale, M. C. (1978). *Basic human needs.* New Brunswick, NJ: Transaction Books.

Meleis, A. I. (1991). *Theoretical nursing: Development and progress* (2nd ed.). New York: Lippincott.

Minshull, J., Ross, K., & Turner, J. (1986). The human needs model of nursing. *Journal of Advanced Nursing, 11,* 643–649.

Montagu, A. (1966). *On being human.* New York: Hawthorn Books.

Montagu, M. F. A. (1955). *The direction of human development: Biological and social bases.* New York: Harper & Brothers.

See, E. M. (1989). Abdellah's model of nursing: Twenty-one nursing problems. In J. J. Fitzpatric & A. L. Whall (Eds.), *Conceptual models of nursing: Analysis and application* (2nd ed., pp. 123–136). Norwalk, CT: Appleton & Lange.

Sites, P. (1992). Human needs and control: A foundation for human science and critique. In R. H. Brown (Ed.), *Writing the social text: Poetics and politics in social science discourse* (pp. 177–197). New York: Aldine Gruyter.

Turner, J. H. (1987). Toward a sociological theory of motivation. *American Sociological Review, 52,* 15–27.

Turner, J. H. (1991a). Microtheorizing. In J. H. Turner (Ed.), *The structure of sociological theory* (5th ed., pp. 592–606). Belmont, CA: Wadsworth Publishing.

Turner, J. H. (1991b). The emergence of functionalism. In J. H. Turner (Ed.), *The structure of sociological theory* (5th ed., pp. 33–50). Belmont, CA: Wadsworth.

Watt, E. D. (1996). Human needs. In A. Kuper & J. Kuper (Eds.), *The social science encyclopedia* (2nd ed., pp. 383–384). New York: Routledge.

Wrightsman, L. S. (1992). *Assumptions about human nature: Implications for researchers and practitioners* (2nd ed.). Newbury Park, CA: Sage.

Yura, H., & Walsh, M. B. (Eds.). (1978). *Human needs and the nursing process.* New York: Appleton-Century-Crofts.

Yura, H., & Walsh, M. B. (1988). *The nursing process: Assessing, planning, implementing, evaluating* (5th ed.). Norwalk, CT: Appleton & Lange.

4

Applying the Concept of Need to Patient Empowerment

Penny Powers

This chapter picks up its central argument from the question left unanswered in the previous chapter regarding the implication of conceptualizing human needs as universal versus socially and politically determined. A postmodern discourse analysis is offered here to examine nursing's conceptualization of human needs and nursing practice framed within such conceptualizations.

Most people could probably provide a definition of the word *need* in their native language. Nursing discourse, however, following psychology (Maslow, 1954; 1970) has used the word need as a concept, a technical and theoretical term that has played an important role in nursing theory and practice beginning with Peplau (1952). Nursing discourse concerning the concept of need is often referred to in the plural form "needs" in an attempt to move away from the medical model of disease. A discipline-specific concept, however, possesses defining attributes, empirical referents, antecedents, and consequences (Walker & Avant, 1988). As a concept in nursing discourse, need functions as an abstract linguistic entity apart from patient situations in specific ways: (a) to organize discourse presented to nursing students about what it means to be a human being, (b) to provide a framework for organizing nursing interventions, and (c) to inform the way we think about nursing as a profession and its role in the social world.

This elevation of the word need to a technical term has proceeded without a formal definition, a concept analysis or examination of the philosophical implications of using the word as a concept. Without these considerations, the concept of need has become taken for granted in nursing. The concept of need is found in many different contexts in nursing literature concerning practice, education, and theory, whereas its use in the discipline of psychology has markedly decreased.

It is the purpose of this chapter to provide one possible discourse analysis of the current status of the concept of need in nursing. Philosophical analysis provides important contributions to theoretical discourse in our discipline (Allen, 1986; Dzurec, 1989; Thompson, 1987). Smith, who has written a philosophical analysis of the concept of health (1981) states "The method of testing ideas in philosophic inquiry is that of critical discussion. . . . The major difference between philosophical inquiry and empirical science is that experiments are not performed in philosophic inquiry" (p. 43). The concept of need is a good candidate for philosophical analysis to initiate discussion concerning its significance, relevance, and the consequences of its use. This analysis does not presume that there is some essential nature to the word or the concept to be uncovered, discovered, invented, or proposed. Instead, it is emphasized that there is an important history to the concept of need that informs the manner in which it is currently used in nursing.

It is the claim of this analysis that the use of the concept of need in nursing has philosophical implications that conflict with generally accepted goals of nursing. More specifically, this analysis claims that the way we as nurses use the concept, (a) assumes that the standards or criteria used for judging the existence and relative weight of need statements are universally applicable to all people at all times (e.g., all prostatectomy patients need continuous urinary irrigation), (b) reflects a view of nursing's relationship to people that limits the autonomy and responsibility of both the nurse and the patient by severely limiting participation in the discourse to experts, (c) contributes to and reproduces an oppressive notion of the role of science and social agency in society, and (d) directs attention away from, or masks, important issues such as sexism, racism, power, knowledge, political action, and human emancipation.

The use of the concept of need without philosophical analysis results in unintended consequences such as the reproduction of social situations that contradict currently accepted ideals and aims of nursing. These contradictions can cause tension in the practice of a discipline (Giddens, 1979). The use of a Foucaultian perspective delineates the historical features of the concept and explains its use as an example of an oppressive discourse in Western society. Examining unintended consequences in this way provides a perspective for exposing discrepancies and explaining tensions within nursing discourse and practice.

THE WORD 'NEED' AND NEED CLAIMS

The derivation, development and refinement of the word need provides the starting point for this analysis (Powers, 1989). The root of the English word comes from old Teutonic and means violence, force, or constraint by or on persons, as "I chopped the wood with need" (forcefully). Indeed, one old form of the word was needforce, but this usage is now considered obsolete (Oxford, 1971). However, force is still detectable in modern synonym discussions in which the emotional force implied by the word need is in contrast with the more formal word, necessity (Webster, 1964). In the oldest use, the associated physical force was plainly visible between one person and another or between a person and an object. The most noticeable change in the evolution of the word for this analysis is that the location and direction of the force has been moved from outside a person to within a person. The only remaining vestige of compulsion is an emotional attachment to our opinion that we need something. We feel compelled instead of being compelled. For example the following sentence demonstrates the emotional attachment to the opinion, "I really need to get out there and pull those weeds out of my garden before they choke out my vegetable seedlings."

Need statements in modern English can be expressed on your own behalf, such as "I need a drink of water" or on behalf of someone else, such as "You need to lose 40 pounds" or for something else, such as "That house needs a fresh coat of paint." Need statements can also be implied by actions. For example, we assume that you change the baby's diapers because they need changing, without saying so unless you are asked. If you are asked for a reason, you often respond with a need statement.

The modern word need no longer refers to externally applied force. It refers instead to an opinion about a compelling relationship to something. This opinion is identified by a socially proper linguistic expression, or implied in an action that is justified by a socially proper linguistic expression. "I need to stop and get some gas. The needle is sitting on 'E'."

It is important to emphasize that the need is the statement, not a physical condition, even when the statement is referring to something associated with a physical condition such as the empty gas tank as referred to above. There is no physical condition of the gas tank that indicates need. The need is the statement by a person. The philosophical debate on this point continues, but the direction is clear (Michalos, 1988; Willard, 1987). All need statements are (explicitly or implicitly) *in order to* statements. That is, they are goal statements. Whenever a need statement is expressed, someone can always ask, "Why do you need that?" "I need some gas if we're going to make it to my sister's place." "I need a drink of water to quench my thirst." "You need to lose 40 pounds in order to get your diabetes under control." "You need two units of blood to stay alive." "That house needs a coat of paint to look attractive." "The baby's diapers needed changing in order to keep her bottom dry." Sometimes, the answers are self-evident, and the in order to justification is implied: "I need a drink of water because I'm thirsty. Why else would I say that?" Since need statements are assertions, there can be disagreement, even in the self-evident case: "I don't know, I thought maybe you needed some water to rinse your mouth, not because you were thirsty."

Fraser (1989) calls these self-evident cases *thin* need statements. They aren't called *needs*, but *need statements*, in order to emphasize the linguistic nature of our understanding of need. Need statements about food, water, and shelter are thin need statements that have self-evident, unexpressed in order to components. On the other hand, the *thick* need statements are not self-evident cases and are normally accompanied by in order to justification clauses. New clothes, a nice house, good food are examples of thick need statements. "I need a new pair of shoes that have Velcro instead of laces because my arthritic fingers can't do laces anymore without a lot of pain."

Need statements are in a form of argument. Need statements, or in order to statements are examples of claim-grounds statements (Toulmin, Reike, & Janik, 1984). It is your claim that you need something, or that your patient needs something, or that the house needs something, and the in order to part of the statement constitutes the grounds (or reasons, or evidence) given to support your claim. In the self-evident cases (the thin need statements) there probably won't be much disagreement, even though there can be. In the drink of water case, for example, I claim I need a drink of water and I give the grounds that I am thirsty. A listener may disagree with the claim that I need a drink of water, but cannot dispute my evidence that I am thirsty.

In the thick need statements, there is more often disagreement. Your claim can be disputed by challenging it with a counter-claim complete with its own grounds or by questioning whether your grounds actually do function to support your claim ("You may feel thirsty, but you do not need a drink of water because your body is over-hydrated as it is."). In the terms of informal logic, this latter challenge is one about *warrants*. A warrant is the statement that asserts the relevance of the grounds to the claim. A warrant is what shows that these grounds do support this claim. A warrant can be implicit or explicit, empirical or ethical, personal or social, depending on the type of claim. With the thin need claims, you usually don't provide a warrant unless you are specifically asked for it.

In the thin need statements, you don't usually supply grounds, much less a warrant, because the warrants as well as the grounds are implicit and usually self-evident. The sarcastic tone of the following sentence implies that the listener must be awfully dense to ask for justification for the claim that someone needs a drink of water: "I need a drink of water {claim} because I'm thirsty! {grounds} People do actually die from dehydration {warrant}, you know!" Thus a common warrant for thin need claims is that it is a good thing for person *x* to have *y*, or for *x* to have *y* now. Need claims are social/linguistic constructions based on assumptions about what human life consists of, including the social standards by which we judge goodness and rightness. The thick need statements, besides being more often asked for grounds, are more often asked for warrants "I need new shoes with Velcro fasteners {claim} because my fingers hurt when I tie laces {grounds}. My fingers don't hurt when I use Velcro fasteners" {warrant}.

Need claims can be further differentiated from other types of claims that people make. This differentiation is demonstrated by the fact that need is subject to different social criteria for evaluation than other kinds of claims, or arguments. Want statements, for example, are also claims, but the social/linguistic criteria for their evaluation are different from the social/linguistic criteria for the evaluation of need claims. When you say you want something, you can always be asked for your grounds in the same manner as a need statement is questioned. In other words, you can be asked, "Why do you want that?" It is acceptable, however, in the case of a want claim, to either provide grounds, or to refuse to provide grounds:

"I want some broccoli."
"Why?"
"I don't know, I just want broccoli, okay?"

The above would not be an acceptable response to a need statement. A need statement requires the in order to justification, and it is acceptable to ask the speaker for the grounds if it is not self-evident:

"I need broccoli."
"Why?"
"I just need broccoli, okay?"
"Come on, you have to have a reason to say you need broccoli."

"I need broccoli because I don't eat dairy products and so I get calcium from broccoli."

"Oh, okay. Now I understand why you need broccoli."

Want statements, therefore, cannot be disputed in the same way as need statements. You can ask for the grounds (the reasons) and you can question the speakers' judgment or their sanity, but you cannot argue the claim. If they want it, they want it. You can say why you wouldn't want it, or you can say why they shouldn't want it, but you can't say "You don't want that," unless you are: (a) questioning their honesty (e.g., "You don't really want a drink of water, you're just trying to postpone going to bed.") or (b) teaching a child how to differentiate between want statements and need statements:

"I don't want a bath"
"Maybe not, but you sure do need a bath"
"I need a cookie"
"No, you want a cookie, but you sure don't need one."

Since our understanding of need is based on social/linguistic relationships (need claims), and these claims are not the same kind of thing as want claims, what kind of claims are they? Claims about need are examples of what Kuhn (1970) and Bernstein (1983) call judgmental statements. Bernstein distinguishes judgmental claims from subjective claims by saying that subjective claims cannot be disputed (i.e., "I really liked that movie") short of the accusation of dishonesty or deceit. Judgmental claims, however, can be subject to dispute (e.g., "That movie was awful.") and are judged by their support, that is, their grounds and warrants. Objective claims, on the other hand, (e.g., "That movie was filmed in Tanzania.") are judged by appeal to objective criteria.

Need claims, therefore, belong in the judgmental category, and want claims are in the subjective category. Need claims always have supporting grounds and warrants, either explicit or implicit. This is to say that need claims are just as rational as objective claims. Such judgmental reasoning is often maligned as "unscientific" or "subjective" because of the acceptability of ethical warrants as support (Bernstein, 1983) and the possibility of counter-claims. Judgmental claims are more clearly judged by standards of social acceptability, not by so-called objective criteria, which, in many views, are also socially defined.

In summary, the following points have been supported: (a) in the evolution of the word need, the location of force has changed from an external visible compulsion to internal emotional force of compelling argument; (b) need statements are claims, that is, a form of argument, subject to social/linguistic evaluation; (c) need claims are subject to different social criteria with respect to their evaluation from other forms of argument, such as want claims, by virtue of the contrasting warrants that are socially/linguistically acceptable. These social standards undergo continuous evolution (Foucault, 1980) as do all social criteria.

THE CONCEPT OF NEED IN NURSING

The concept of need has been utilized widely in nursing theory and practice. Such an influential concept should receive scrutiny of its history, discourse, implications, and assumptions. The concept of need has a negative orientation among some nursing theorists because it reinforces a continued emphasis on human deficits (Meleis, 1985) that mirrors the biomedical deficit treatment model. Several early nursing theories have been characterized as need theories, but the concept itself was not defined by any of these authors (Meleis, 1985). In this category, Meleis includes Peplau, Henderson, and among more recent authors, Abdellah and Orem (Meleis, 1985). The work of psychologist Abraham Maslow (1954, 1970) is an important foundation for these of all theorists, especially for Peplau, who can be considered the main source of influence for Maslow's work in nursing (Peplau, 1952).

Nursing need theories were developed in answer to the functional question, What do nurses do? The answer for these theorists was, nurses meet or help patients to meet needs. The need theories focus on problems, take a reductionist approach to human beings as a set of problems, and nursing to a set of controlling functions (Meleis, 1985, p. 172). These early theories portray nurses as the decision makers in the care process, and do not address the perception of the client, a view of the environment, or a process of interaction (Meleis, 1985, p. 172).

It is interesting to note that these theories are considered by some to be outdated foundational influences, and yet these assumptions continue to inform nursing literature. There have been several more recent works that propose or apply an existing human need model (Ellis & Nowlis, 1994; Minshull, Ross, & Turner, 1986). Lilley (1987), for example, has developed the Human Needs Assessment Scale based on Yura and Walsh (1983).

Interestingly, Maslow's work lacks a definition of need and also lacks any concept of a hierarchy of needs (1954, 1970). Yura and Walsh (1983) have defined the concept of need more recently in nursing, however, as an objectively measurable internal tension resulting from an alteration in the individual. This definition reflects assumptions that have been discredited in philosophical literature. There is no adequate evidence for assuming the existence of a physically detectable internal tension from a verbal statement of need (Michalos, 1988). Furthermore, this definition of need as an internal tension reifies a social/linguistic concept into a physical entity; locates the entity within individuals; and charges nurses to identify, name, and treat the condition. The goal of treatment is to eliminate the assumed alteration causing the tension. This process completely strips the social/linguistic, personal, and interactive nature of need identification to produce a science of needs. Nurses become the social agents of the resulting scientific body of knowledge that describes the alterations and the tensions, prescribes the treatments, and judges the outcomes by prescribed measurable criteria.

SOCIAL AGENTS OF NEED

The choice of a role for nurses of assessing and treating needs contains serious unexamined assumptions with regard to the notion of social agency (Allen, 1987). Nursing literature has not specifically addressed the philosophical notion of nurses as agents of social order. Social agents include such categories as teachers, police, bureaucrats, professionals, and other rule-enforcing authority figures that possess distinct bodies of knowledge about people and the social authority to do something about it. Social agents have always held higher status than occupations without such power/knowledge. According to Michel Foucault (1965, 1975, & 1980), the notion of social agents (which he sometimes called disciplinary technologists to emphasize the technical role) has become an important consideration in modern discussions of power because of the large amount of knowledge, power, and practices that have been developed in the social sciences. The training of social agents in each of the new areas of the human sciences has become widely institutionalized, and acceptance of this category of person has become unquestioned.

The assumption of the acceptability of power and control over others for their own good is an explicit part of our education as nurses. For example, we are educated that science is an everevolving process toward truths that give social agents the tools to predict and control outcomes that facilitate the advancement of civilization and are therefore desirable. Academics produce the research that guides the practice that supports the research, which benefits society as a whole.

Nursing has a long-standing goal of increased power and influence in the social world based on models from other professions. As another category of social agents, nurses have as part of that role the task of the revelation and enforcement of the normalized truths of their own brand of social science for the assumed order and benefit of all. Foucault presents compelling arguments to demonstrate that research in the social sciences is a powerful force for expanding the prediction and control of finer and finer details of people's lives (Foucault, 1980). The statistical average often becomes the enforced normal. Foucault claims that people in Western civilization have generally come to accept the importance of the role of social agents (Foucault, 1979).

People have internalized the importance of being measured, examined, and compared to a standard, to the point that they compare themselves to published standards such as height/weight tables, normal blood pressure charts, or stages of grief. This large-scale social process results in social control of internal compulsions at all levels, from production to justification to expression (Dreyfus & Rabinow, 1983). This process is clearly reflected in the historic evolution of the word need. Need statements have been redefined as an internal tension and made subject to diagnosis and treatment by a social agent using criteria that have been normalized from scientific averages. Patients are socialized to understand under what circumstances it is permissible for the claims of an individual to be overruled by a professional armed with a normal curve, scientific truth, and a nursing intervention.

The science of need gives members of society who are trained social agents the responsibility of enforcing dominant ideologies of the culture in which they have been carefully educated. One of the dominant ideologies in our Western society is male-centered, power-based, empirical analytic science, which carries the assumptions of the value of efficiency, standardization, prediction, and control (Powers, 1992). If an individual does not conform to the influence of the dominant ideologies through social agents, the blame then falls on the individual, not on the science or the social agent. In this case, the problem lies within the person and that person's faulty socialization process, or lack of compliance. Furthermore, people accept this blame, when it is affixed by social agents supported by the vast power/knowledge of science, because science is a very powerful model.

We as nurses readily accept the role of social agent based on social science without a philosophical analysis of the historical antecedents and present consequences of our position. This renders impossible a conscious decision concerning whether to acknowledge and participate in the process of extending the practices of prediction and control to newly defined subject areas in human life without acknowledging the social/linguistic nature of need claims made by embodied, situated speakers.

Nursing discourses include goals concerning patient advocacy, collaboration in decision making, patient teaching, patient perspective, environmental influences, cultural sensitivity, critical thinking, conflict resolution, and other so-called empowering strategies and perspectives. On the other hand, nursing actions based on the concept of need perpetuate the acceptability of oppression through scientific prediction and control (Meleis, 1985) using justifications phrased in terms of patient outcomes that are deceptive to both patients and nurses.

Nursing research on interventions is aimed at outcome measures such as compliance and normal responses (Iowa Intervention Project, 1993). We use our discourse to construct the patient conditions that we diagnose, the treatments that we administer, and the units of measurement for the outcomes we seek; all in terms of normalized truth that has been standardized by research (Carpenito, 1995). Patient teaching, for example, resembles oppression more than learning, with the emphasis on outcomes instead of understanding. This approach to the nurse/patient encounter assumes that it is in the interests of society to produce outcomes, instead of fostering understanding from the patient perspective. We assume that the problems in patient compliance can be overcome with more science, more research, into more interventions that produce better outcomes.

ALTERNATIVE FUTURES FOR NURSING DISCOURSE ON NEED

Nursing literature has recently begun to address such topics as power and oppression. Allen and colleagues suggest that research about the conduct of research would be extremely useful in this regard (Allen, Allman, & Powers, 1991). Sawicki suggests a "politics of difference" for nursing literature (1986). Thompson suggests critical scholarship as an approach to the critique of domination in nursing (1987). Hall, Stevens, and Meleis (1994) discuss the concept of marginalization. Mason and colleagues (1994) address the empowering results of education for staff nurses. A critical social theory perspective of political agendas is examined by Dickerson and Campbell-Heider (1994). None of these discussions has a focus on the concept of need. There are, however, some relevant writings in postmodern feminist theory.

Fraser, for example, suggests that emphasis be shifted to a discourse about need identifications instead of need satisfactions (Fraser, 1989).

The importance of this distinction lies in the fact that restricting talk to need satisfactions assumes that the nature of the concept of needs is unproblematic in the first place. Shifting talk away from need satisfaction to need identification is important because the former assumes that all needs are universal human qualities that are already identified and agreed on, that is, they have assumed warrants for their expression in our social world.

Restricting dialogue to need satisfactions obscures the politically contestable nature of both thin and thick need statements. Thus, at first glance it may seem obvious that people need housing, but it is not so apparent as to what kind of housing people need and how it is acceptable to go about getting it, or be given it, or to take it. Talk about need identification, however, directs attention to the specifics of who decides what the need is and what grounds and warrants are acceptable supports for the need claims. Talk about need identification amounts to letting people construct their own arguments for their need claims, to be communicatively achieved in an overtly political social world. This type of dialogue does not assume the existence of universal scientifically normalized needs whose satisfaction is assessed and prescribed by social agents. One effect of such a shift may be to emphasize understanding and negotiation instead of outcomes.

Fraser also notes that restricting talk about need to talk about need satisfaction instead of need identification also serves the purpose of bypassing discussion concerning the possibility that the process of need identification is in itself oppressive and favors dominant groups in the social world. Discourse in the social sciences concerning need satisfaction is thus restricted to norm-discovering, statistical, empirical analytic methodology, which has been described as necessarily resulting in oppression of subordinate groups (Foucault, 1979).

Fraser uses the concept of need specifically in this context to illustrate how a dominant ideology can co-opt a nondominant discourse, bypassing talk about the nature of need and instead talking about the distribution of need satisfactions. Foucault calls this process "the medicalization of social control" (O'Neill, 1986) because this kind of talk takes social/ethical discourse and turns it into a technical problem to be solved by social agents using normalized scientific truths. Medicalization of social control removes the inherently political nature of need identification from the discussion and creates new fields for social science and the education of new forms of social agents at the same time.

Talk about need and talk about rights have been described as characteristic of our form of late welfare capitalism (Fraser, 1989). From a Foucaultian perspective this is to say that the only socially acceptable warrants for need claims in late welfare capitalist discourse are those that are constructed on the basis of social science, thus limiting participation in the discussion to those social agents educated to understand science. This process effectively eliminates talk about need identification by situated individuals who may or may not understand how science works. Instead, talk is limited to scientific discussion concerning the distribution of need satisfactions based on principles of welfare capitalism. Dreyfus and Rabinow say explicitly, "The administrative apparatus of the state posed welfare in terms of people's needs and happiness" (Dreyfus & Rabinow, 1983, p. 139).

When people are acknowledged to have rights, there is an assumed definition of the good life, or what it is to which people have rights. This definition provides the grounds and warrants for need goal statements, such that "I need *x* in order to get *y*," *y* being something to which you have a right. Oppressed groups are linguistically/scientifically acknowledged to have the same rights as everyone else, but can nevertheless experience discrimination. A group can be acknowledged to have a right to something, acknowledged to have a right to state the need to get it, but not acknowledged to have the right to access the means to get it. Similarly, other groups of people are simply not acknowledged socially to fit the definition of a person who has these rights or only acknowledged to have the right to a lesser quality of that something. Furthermore, subordinate groups tend to internalize these conditions as normal and unquestioned (Friere, 1972).

Two examples illustrate this form of oppression. First, consider that groups of citizens find it difficult to make a case to define their need for medical care in terms of care that does not discriminate against them on the basis of some social/linguistic category such as race. This difficulty arises from the fact that the need for medical care is already defined without reference to race by the hegemonic influence of medical discourse. The only case that it is possible to make is one that refers to the distribution of medical care as it has already been defined. Even then, a redefinition of, say, illegal aliens as not citizens effectively rules out their participation in the discourse. This move serves to retain the philosophical definition of needs to include their universal application to all humans, but removes illegal aliens from the category of human beings, thus denying them both the services and participation in the discussion.

Secondly, consider that discourse concerning the distribution of need satisfaction for scientifically normalized needs supports an illusion of choices. Thinking that we have rights to need satisfaction gives an illusion of autonomy. Instead, autonomous choices are severely limited because our needs are not self-defined. Instead, need has already been defined by the scientific research process instead of the process of political discourse.

Thus, autonomy is restricted to choices among methods of need satisfaction that may be wholly unsatisfactory or completely closed to that individual. Accordingly, you as an immigrant can assume that you have a right to the good life and still find that you have no right to the means to get it (Willard, 1987) and be completely at a loss to understand how to object to the manner in which this happened.

As nurses, we give patients illusions of choice that allow them to assume the right to have the choice implemented. At the same time, we sometimes deny the definition of person to someone, say, with a mental illness, or deny someone access to the means to get their need met because of the cost of advice concerning how to do it. This is part of the role of social agents because the general outcomes of research assume more importance than a single case.

Nurses are in a position to feel conflict between the assumptions of a trained social agent and the position of a member of an oppressed group because nursing is traditionally a female occupation and at the same time presents itself as based on scientific research. The continually shifting dominant and subordinate relationships can cause tension within the practice of nursing. To patients we are dominant. To physicians and hospital administrators nurses are subordinate. To the lay public we are dominant. A nurse may be faced with trying to advocate with medicine for a patient, while at the same time trying to advocate for medicine to the patient and uphold some degree of professionalism. This tension within nursing practice causes horizontal classism and racism within the discipline because of the self-deprecation that comes with oppressed group behavior (Friere, 1972; Roberts, 1983).

Goals of nursing such as found in the American Nursing Association's Social Policy Statement have received careful critique (Allen, 1987). One key goal of the discipline of nursing is professionalization based partly on the criterion of the acquisition of a scientific body of knowledge and phrased in terms of people's needs, happiness, and health (Gamer, 1979). This goal reflects a desire among nurses for increased social power, prestige, and control. Based on the models from other professions, the goal requires an independent body of scientific knowledge that affords prediction and control of outcomes specific to the discipline. To this end, nursing has tried to ally with professional groups who achieved status on the basis of exclusion, rather than empowerment (O'Neill, 1991).

Professionalism in these terms would mean the loss of perspectives from working-class nurses and nurses of color. In addition, nursing would remove itself from the strengths available from the discourses of unionism and feminism. The loss of these discourses would restrict available subject positions from which nurses could speak in terms of need identification. Furthermore, professionalization in these terms would limit the possibility of discourses in nursing that are not based on traditional social science.

CONCLUSIONS

The concept of needs in nursing is a top-down, mechanistic, means-end, product-oriented list of technical functions for nurses in a role of social agency where the major goal is patient compliance with predetermined scientific categories. The process of assessing and treating need avoids revealing previously formed value decisions made without mutual consent of individual patients and enforced without discussion. The warrants that provide the justification for this approach are efficiency, advancing scientific method, professionalization, and standardization.

The following recommendations for nursing arise from this discussion. Teaching nursing students the concept of need, in a list or a hierarchy, reinforces the assumption that needs are reified physical entities to be measured, diagnosed, and treated. We should instead emphasize talk about need statements as claims made by embodied, situated speakers, supported by grounds, and warrants that mean something in the context of the lives of speaker and listener. Nurses can encourage a person's ability to determine and support their own need claims, even if it contradicts our own. The concept of collaboration is lost when the underlying assumption of nurse as social agent places so much weight on the ideal of compliance.

Students might well benefit from an appreciation of our position as patient advocates as well as a revised concept of social agency. These perspectives offer us opportunities apart from traditional professional goals.

Nurses can produce their own arguments, their own claims, grounds and warrants in an arena of public discourse (Thompson, 1987). There is an argument to be made for nursing not as a science, but as a practical-moral way of being in the world (Yarling & McElmurry, 1986) that entails practical reasoning and informed judgment. New to academia, the discipline of nursing has the opportunity to demonstrate the operation of a practice discipline informed by many interrelated bodies of knowledge including its own widely varying discourses in service to communicably achieved moral ideals through the efforts of situated human beings. It would be difficult to estimate the consequences, both intended and unintended, of the concept of needs on nursing at this point in its history. Although nursing practice has long been informed by this concept, further analysis of the discourse of needs seems warranted.

REFERENCES

Allen, D. (1986). Using philosophical and historical methodologies to understand the concept of health. In P. Chinn (Ed.), *Nursing research methodology* (pp. 157–168). Rockville, MD: Aspen.

Allen, D. (1987). The social policy statement: A reappraisal. *Advances in Nursing Science, 10,* 39–48.

Allen, D., Allman, K., & Powers, P. (1991). Feminist research without gender. *Advances in Nursing Science, 13,* 49.

Bernstein, R. (1983). *Beyond Objectivism and Relativism: Science, Hermeneutics and Praxis.* Philadelphia: University of Pennsylvania Press.

Carpenito, L. J. (1995). *Nursing Diagnosis: Application to Clinical Practice, Sixth Edition.* Philadelphia: Lippincott.

Dickerson, S. S., & Campbell-Heider, N. (1994). Interpreting political agendas from a critical social theory perspective. *Nursing Outlook, 42,* 265–271.

Dreyfus, H., & Rabinow, P. (1983). *Michel Foucault, Beyond Structuralism and Hermeneutics.* Chicago: University of Chicago Press.

Dzurec, L. (1989). The necessity for and evolution of multiple paradigms for nursing research: A poststructuralist perspective. *Advances in Nursing Science, 11,* 69–77.

Ellis, J. R., & Nowlis, E. A. (1994). *Nursing: A human needs approach* 5th ed. Hagerstown, MD: Lippincott.

Foucault, M. (1965). *Madness and civilization* (R. Howard, Trans.). New York: Vintage/Random House. (Original work published in 1961.)

Foucault, M. (1975). *The birth of the clinic* (A. M. Sheridan Smith, Trans.). New York: Vintage/Random House. (Original work published in 1963.)

Foucault, M. (1979). *Discipline and punish: The birth of the prison* (A. Sheridan, Trans.). New York: Vintage/Random House. (Original work published in 1975.)

Foucault, M. (1980). *The history of sexuality* (Vol. 1–3). (R. Hurley, Trans.). New York: Random House. (Original work published in 1976.)

Fraser, N. (1989). *Unruly Practices: Power, Discourse and Gender in Contemporary Social Theory.* Minneapolis, MN: University of Minnesota Press.

Friere, P. (1972). *Pedagogy of the oppressed* (pp. 20–28). New York: Penguin.

Gamer, M. (1979). The Ideology of professionalism. *Nursing Outlook, 27,* 108–111.

Giddens, A. (1979). *Central Problems in Social Theory.* London: Macmillan.

Hall, J. M., Stevens, P. E., & Meleis, A. I. (1994). Marginalization: A guiding concept for valuing diversity in nursing knowledge. *Advances in Nursing Science, 16,* 23–41.

Iowa Intervention Project. (1993). *NIC Interventions Linked to NANDA Diagnoses.* Iowa City, IA: Iowa Intervention Project.

Kuhn, T. (1970). *The structure of scientific revolutions* (2nd ed.). Chicago: University of Chicago Press.

Lilley, L. (1987). Human need fulfillment alteration in the client with uterine cancer. *Cancer Nursing, 10,* 327–337.

Maslow, A. (1954 & 1970). *Motivation and personality* (1st & 2nd eds.). New York: Harper and Row.

Mason, D. J., Costello-Nickitas, D. M., Scanlan, J. M., & Magnuson, B. A. (1994). Empowering nurses for politically astute change in the workplace. *Journal of Continuing Education in Nursing, 22,* 5–10.

Meleis, A. (1985). *Theoretical nursing: Development and progress.* Philadelphia: Lippincott.

Michalos, A. (1988). Meeting current needs. *Dialogue, 27,* 507–515.

Minshull, J., Ross, K., & Turner, J. (1986). The human needs model of nursing. *Journal of Advanced Nursing, 11,* 643–649.

O'Neill, J. (1986). The medicalization of social control. *Canadian Review of Sociology and Anthropology, 23,* 350–364.

O'Neill, S. (1991). *The drive for professionalism in Nursing: A reflection of classism and racism.* Paper presented at the Critical Theory and Feminist Theory in Nursing Conference, Toledo, Ohio.

Oxford English Dictionary (Compact Edition). (1971). London: Oxford University Press.

Peplau, H. (1952). *Interpersonal relations in nursing.* New York: Putnam.

Powers, P. (1989). *Needs—A concept analysis.* Unpublished manuscript.

Powers, P. (1992). *Needs in nursing.* Unpublished master's thesis. University of Washington, Seattle, WA.

Roberts, S. (1983). Oppressed group behavior: Implications for nursing. *Advances in Nursing Science, 6,* 21–30.

Sawicki, J. (1986). Foucault and feminism: Toward a politics of difference. *Hypatia, 1,* 23–36.

Thompson, J. (1987). Critical scholarship: The critique of domination in nursing. *Advances in Nursing Science, 10,* 27–38.

Toulmin, S., Reike, R., & Janik, A. (1984) *An introduction to reasoning* (2nd ed.). New York: MacMillan.

Walker, L., & Avant, K. (1988). *Strategies for theory construction in nursing* (2nd ed.). Norwalk, CT: Appleton and Lange.

Webster's New World Dictionary. (1964). New York: World.

Willard, L. (1987). Needs and rights. *Dialogue, 26,* 43–53.

Yarling, R., & McElmurry, B. (1986). The moral foundation of nursing. *Advances in Nursing Science, 8,* 63–73.

Yura, H., & Walsh, M. B. (1983). *The nursing process: Assessment, planning, implementing, evaluating* (3rd ed.). New York: Appleton-Century-Crofts.

5

The Concept of Interaction in Theory and Practice*

Susanne Wied

In the field of nursing and caring the term *interaction* is used in an exceedingly vague manner. There are three basic concepts from which to choose. I examine in the first, theoretical, in which no claim is made to any exhaustive treatment of the term's usage. My aim, rather, is to look into and clarify aspects of the notion of interaction, which are relevant to nursing in both theory and practice.

Interaction has much to do with language. Today, it is scarcely possible to separate the term from the notion of communication, and also the written word constitutes a form of communication within the system of nursing and caring.

In this contribution I confine my considerations to interaction between people. However, I would add that, if one were to discard the psychosocial conceptualization of the term, it would be equally rewarding and important to examine interaction between fields or systems. Here, however, we would be moving onto a different plane of the notion of interaction, which would lead us to an abstract, epistemological discussion of the subject. Once there is greater acceptance of the theoretical side of nursing, there will certainly be an occasion for such a discussion; for the moment, however, it would no doubt merely produce "contemporary esoteric 'episto' babble" (Guttman, 1990, p. 148). Of greater consequence at present, in my view, is the practice-oriented use and application of fundamental psychological, humanistic, and sociological concepts in the context of nursing and caring.

*Translated from German by Gerald Nixon.

In the *Duden Book of Loanwords* (1982) the term interaction is defined as "actions relating to each other of two or more persons" and "reciprocal relationships between partners." The term is regarded as belonging to the fields of sociology and psychology. In Fuchs-Heinritz's *Dictionary of Sociology* (1994) interaction is first defined in the plain sense of its Latin source as "reciprocal effect," before being divided into its manifold meanings; and among these a special place is given to "social interaction." According to the sociologist Talcott Parsons (1949), interaction denotes the social actions performed between two people (ego and alter). The actions are reciprocally oriented toward fulfilling the expectations of the other. Interaction is bound to social roles and governed by common regulative norms. In the work of the social psychologist George Herbert Mead (1934), the focus is placed on the actions of partners performed through symbols, which have the same meaning for both partners. Basing his assumptions on his ethnographic studies, Goffman (1967) distinguishes between centered and noncentered interaction. Here, the attention of the partners is directed toward common points of reference (e.g., social occasions); the partners cooperate to maintain these points of reference and, if they are jeopardized, negative sanctions are imposed. Otherwise, in accumulating information, the interactants concentrate on their perception of each other. Watzlawick and coauthors in their Pragmatics of Human Communication (1967) consider interaction from the perspective of communication theory and defined it systemically as the sending and receiving of messages between two or more persons. I will return to this theoretical approach at a later point.

In its colloquial usage the term interaction is heard when topics take a psycho-sociological or sociopsychological turn—although, in effect, it is nebulously used in the plain sense of the mutual effects of whatever two things come into contact with each other. In the *Dictionary of Psychiatry and Medical Psychology* (Wörterbuch der Psychiatrie . . . , 1977), interaction is defined as "a kind of mutual relationship between the members of a group . . . ," although it is not made clear whether it applies to the relationship between the individuals or between their messages. The interpretation is left to the reader. It is this very lack of clarity in the notion of relationship that causes difficulty as does the diffuse nature of the notion of interaction. When we talk about interaction, we are not writing, speaking, reading, or thinking about the same thing; as Mead would put it, we are not basing the linguistic symbol interaction on the same meaning.

INTERACTION AND NURSING THEORY

To illustrate my hypothesis of the diffuse usage of the term, I would like to go into closer detail about the views of nursing scholars, such as Meleis, Fawcett, Peplau, King, and Paterson and Zderad on interaction.

Meleis (1991) dates the rise of an interactionist school of thought in nursing to the 1950s and early 1960s. According to her, the theories of this school were centered on the development of a relationship between patient and nurse. They "focused their attention on the process of care and on the ongoing interaction between nurses and clients. Their theories were based on interactionism, phenomenology, and existentialist philosophy" (Meleis, 1991, p. 255). Accordingly, she categorizes the theories proposed by King, Paterson and Zderad, and Peplau as "interaction theories."

King's theory of goal attainment is primarily based on the notion that through transaction between patients and nurses, patients can attain their goals of recovery and health (King, 1981). Similarly, Peplau (1962) proposed that interpersonal relationships between nurses and patients are the processes through which both parties could mature. Paterson and Zderad, on the other hand, viewed people's (that is, patients and nurses) existential connections as the scene through which positive experiences can come about (Paterson & Zderad, 1970/1971, 1988).

In defining the role of nursing Meleis summarizes King's view as a "process of action, reaction, and interaction whereby nurse and client share information about their perceptions of the nursing situation and agree on goals" (1991, p. 256). She also summarizes the definition of interaction by Paterson and Zderad as a "human dialogue, intersubjective transaction, a shared situation, a transactional process, a presence of both patient and nurse" (1991, p. 256). Peplau's definition is summarized by Meleis as a "therapeutic interpersonal, serial, goal-oriented process; a health-focused human relationship" (1991, p. 256).

King puts the focus of nursing on "nurse-patient interactions that lead to goal attainment in a natural environment" (Meleis, 1991, p. 256). Paterson and Zderad, on the other hand, are seen to view the focus of nursing in the sense that the "patient is a unique being; patient's perception of events; both patient and nurse are the focus" (Meleis, 1991, p. 256). For Peplau the focus is on the "nurse-patient relationship and its phases: orientation, identification, exploitation, and resolution; harnessing energy from anxiety and tension to positively defining, understanding, and meeting productively the problem at hand" (Meleis, 1991, p. 256).

According to King the goals of nursing are to "help individuals maintain their health so they can function in their role" (Meleis, 1991, p. 257). While, Paterson and Zderad consider the goals to be to "develop human potential, more well-being for both patient and nurse" (Meleis, 1991, p. 257). On the other hand, Peplau sees them in "develop[ing] personality, making illness an eventful experience; forward movement of personality and other ongoing human processes in the direction of creative, constructive, productive personal and community living" (Meleis, 1991, p. 257).

Problems in nursing arise, according to King, "when nurse and patient do not perceive each other; the situation, or communicate information, transactions are not made, goals are not attained" (Meleis, 1991, p. 257). For Paterson and Zderad problems occur when "people with perceived needs [are] related to the health/illness quality of living," while in Peplau's view, problems are the result of "unsuccessful or incomplete learning of life tasks; energy used in tensions and frustrations due to unmet needs" (Meleis, 1991, p. 257).

Thus, in Meleis' category of interaction theories we are presented with three different theoretical currents. King's approach has its source in the publications of Peplau (and at another point also in Martha Rogers) and in the sociologically oriented studies of interaction of authors like Parsons.

One aspect that does not stand out strongly enough in Meleis' categorization is King's clear orientation toward a systems theory that is expressed in her writings. Indeed, in her further elaboration of interaction theories, Meleis defines the term interaction not from the point of view of communication theory but rather (if at all) from a humanistic standpoint in keeping with the approaches taken by Paterson and Zderad (Meleis, 1991, pp. 258–260). I will return to the differences later.

Peplau's approach, on the other hand, is clearly derived from an analytically oriented psychiatry represented by Sullivan. Peplau has never claimed to have developed her own distinct theory. What she has done is to make the knowledge gained in a psychodynamically oriented psychiatry productive and fruitful for nursing, and this has given utmost clarity to her view of interaction. Here, we are dealing with individuals who have entered a relationship with each other, which can be divided into clear phases and has clear objectives. Interaction is used as an instrument with which to release the potential for development in individuals and initiate processes of learning and maturing. In contrast to the systems approach there is no separation between message, or information, and person; instead, one person is put in relation to another in the concept of transference and countertransference. With regard to nursing we thus have a clear and unequivocal concept of action that can be very well applied to an analytical or psychodynamic setting.

When we move into a systems-oriented or family-oriented context of therapy, whether on the ward or elsewhere, we are drawn into problems of interface because we are mixing two notions of interaction: the relationship approach based on persons and the systems approach based on information, on which a large part of King's theory (1981) is based. Here, however, it is necessary to separate—merely theoretically, of course—the person from the information, or message. The person as a system (which is vigorously disputed among sociologically oriented systems theorists), that is, an individual, exchanges information with another person, resulting in a system of its own, which, detached from the individuals giving the information, constitutes interaction. The exchange of words and gestures in the system family (which King calls the interpersonal system), for example, results in a dynamic process that takes place independently of the participants or, as Watzlawick writes, "once structures of communication have been formed, they develop a life of their own which the individual participants are largely powerless to control" (Watzlawick, 1996, p. 48). These "self-organizing systems" are sometimes more "enduring" than the persons involved—a phenomenon that everyone knows who has enjoyed the peculiar fascination of family get-togethers. The same holds true for what King calls the "social systems" operating in hospitals. Here, patterns of communication continue to exist long after the roles originally allotted have changed. King does not consistently maintain the systems approach in her theory because she would otherwise demand from nurses a considerably greater ability to detach themselves. In regarding interaction as the exchange of information, I keep myself, as a person, as detached as I possibly can from what is taking place and, instead, analyze the wholes of the highly complex and labyrinthine process of communication to contribute to an explanation of as well as a change in the structures. Expressed in terms of the chaos theory, I destroy, in the therapeutic context, old attractors (patterns of order in chaotic vortices) only to establish new ones elsewhere. In the case of radical systems models, for example that of Tschacher, I have no intention—contrary to humanistic or analytical approaches—of bringing myself to bear in my quality as a person and human being. That I nevertheless remain a person and a human being constitutes the informal part of the relationship, not the professional. Here, Tschacher arrives at an important conclusion: "It is quite possible that the new attractor leads to other problems as well as new sufferings. Who is to take responsibility in view of the complex causality of self-organized systems. The desire not to cause harm does not eliminate the risks involved in effective intervention. I fear that ethical notions of responsibility are—at least partially—irreconcilable with systemic thinking since the latter can remain neither centered on the person nor linearly causal" (Tschacher, 1990, p. 162).

In her systems theory King ultimately remains centered on the person, which, unfortunately with regard to interaction, waters down her otherwise sensible and logical approach. She thus defines interaction as a "process of perception and communication between person and person, and person and environment, represented by verbal and nonverbal behaviors that are goal-directed" (Fawcett, 1995, p. 139). This definition remains unclear because of the notion of behavior, which is introduced into it without being defined. And whether interaction is always purpose-oriented is a moot point. Furthermore, we must examine whether it is possible to describe an individual as a personal system without getting into difficulty with perhaps incompatible subsystems within the system human being. I have not yet found any satisfactory answer to this assumption. The counter-hypothesis, put forward for example by Luhmann (1996), that we can equate individuals not with systems but with entities, is far more convincing from the point of view of a systems theory, but it is not possible to elaborate on this here. It must also be borne in mind that in her later writings Martha Rogers no longer speaks of the human being as an open system. However, with a mixed form of personal and informational interaction, which has no conceptual foundation, we are faced with a difficulty concerning the inner logic of King's theoretical edifice. Even though she calls her theory a general systems theory, her assumptions tend to be based on Parson's model of social roles within the system of society.

Paterson and Zderad's humanistic approach presents people in dialogue with each other. It is based explicitly on Carl Rogers' humanistic psychology and on the philosophies of religion drawn up by Buber and Marcel. These two authors choose phenomenology as their method. The key aspect of their notion of nursing is the ability to empathize, although they are at pains to stress that they are talking of a clinical empathy that must be trained and does not lead to the merging of two persons and being one with each other but, through the very ability to detach oneself, is able to create genuine therapeutic closeness (Zderad, 1969, pp. 655–657). What we find here is thus a humanistic rather than a systemic or psychological approach—an approach in which interaction is understood as a deeply sincere and in no way directive encounter between people.

Humanistic and existentialist approaches to nursing enjoy great popularity among German-speaking students of nursing and also among conference participants who come into contact with nursing theory. However, one must not underestimate the dangers lurking in the admirably humane concepts of earlier thinkers. Without adequate training but with great moral goals, people who do not give sufficient reflection to how such methods are to be implemented quickly exhaust themselves. The profound existential and spiritual experience that can be gained in nursing urgently requires the ability to detach oneself. If not, it is possible that the basic concept of nursing is perverted and nurses cling to patients to fill their own empty existence. Unconsciously, they abuse their power in their dealings with the people entrusted to their care or, conversely, they allow themselves to be misused. The goal of maturing together with the patient demanded by humanistic theorists should be regarded with caution. In the writings of Carl Rogers and Martin Buber these goals are expressed with far greater modesty and with less pathos. It may be added that both men were quite aware that they were not true scientists or true philosophers. It is a fundamental, ethical disposition, which brings forth the desire to encounter people without constraints and in a dialogue rather than a scientific model drawn up from humanistic theories. Such a disposition is thus valuable for anyone working in a therapeutic context especially in view of the ethical problems (e.g., systemic thinking) discussed above. Nursing theorists, however, become involved in highly complicated communication structures (systemically expressed) when they present this disposition and this goal as a science in the presence of other scientists.

The question that remains is whether any purpose is served by categorizing such divergent currents of thought under the heading interaction theories. The distinctions are clear enough when one reads Meleis' actual words, but they become greatly obscured in the pedestrian summaries of theory categorizations that have adorned nursing journals for years.

Fawcett's categorization is clearer (1995, p. 20). For her an "interactive approach" has a clear sociological foundation and is bound up with the notions of perception, communication, role, and self-image. She has no use for tabular categorizations of the supposed currents followed by different theorists, merely providing the reader with an overview of categorizations already undertaken by other authors.

Thus, for the context of nursing, no satisfactory definition of the term interaction has yet been found, even if the case studies described by Peplau and Friedemann, for example, lead one to suspect that the authors have indeed drawn up a very clear concept of interaction for themselves.

INTERACTION AND HUMAN COMMUNICATION

Wittgenstein ends his *Tractatus Logico-Philosophicus* with the words: "What we cannot speak about we must pass over in silence" (1997, p.

174). Yet everyday we do the exact opposite and try to express in words and make understandable things that cannot be rendered understandable—the ego to the alter or, as Canetti writes: "How much one must say in order to be heard when one is silent at last" (1976, p. 58).

It would be presumptuous to claim that one wanted to explain such complex phenomena as interaction and communication in a complete and comprehensive manner. Our sense organs are by no means capable of recording all elements and, although retrospective analysis (e.g., video replay) makes us all the wiser with the benefit of hindsight, we still have no chance of achieving this because after the event in a two-dimensional perspective and with changes in sounds and colors we have moved on to another plane, that of communication technology. In spite of this, most people believe that they understand their fellow human beings. There are a few who go insane in order not to have to carry on the business of believing that they understand their fellow human beings. And there are those, too, who, with the aid of such methods as hermeneutics or linguistic and systems analysis, try to pick up and follow the thread that runs through the labyrinth of human communication, thus spending their lives as philosophers, writers, or researchers in the field of communication and—of late—also as nursing theorists.

A quite useful and practicable model for nursing has, in my view, been provided by the research studies undertaken by Watzlawick and colleagues. I would like, therefore, to briefly present the key axioms of this model before turning to nursing practice.

Watzlawick's observation that "one cannot not communicate" has now apparently become an integral part of the repertoire of modern catch phrases such as holistic nursing or maintaining standards. This observation, however, which forms his first pragmatic axiom (Watzlawick, Beaver, & Jackson, 1967, p. 51), is the product of a research study carried out over many years on a solid systems theory basis. At the core of the research is the study of the pragmatics of human communication, the term pragmatics being taken from semiotics (in linguistics the study of signs). The aim of the study was not to seek an explanation for the essence or nature of behavior but to describe the observable manifestations of human relationships. According to Watzlawick, the vehicle of such manifestations is communication (1967, p. 21).

Single acts of communication are called messages; a sequence of reciprocal messages between two or more persons is called interaction. These terms are thus intimately connected with each other.

The material for communication is understood to be every kind of sign, whether verbal or nonverbal, that is, all forms of behavior. As in semiotics, communication is divided into three fields: syntactics, semantics, and pragmatics. Syntactics deals purely with problems of sending and receiving information (codes, redundancy, etc.); semantics has to do with the meaning of message symbols; and pragmatics is concerned with the effects of communication on the behavior of those taking part in it. This division, of course, is purely theoretical, and the three fields are closely interwoven in real-life communication. The study examined the basic features of communication as well as interference in it. Unlike King, Watzlawick does not go as far as to present the reader with an ideal model of communication; instead, especially through his analysis of its interference, he contributes to the possibility of developing more effective tools of understanding. A further observation by Watzlawick also deserves attention. Communication research only has natural language at its disposal, even if it is a question of metacommunication, communication about communication. In contrast to what happens in mathematics, this leads to a lack of precision in formulating messages—a familiar phenomenon to anyone involved in nursing.

His first axiom is a metacommunicational axiom: "One cannot not communicate" (Watzlawick, Beaver, & Jackson, 1967, p. 51). His second axiom is: "Every communication has a content and a relationship aspect such that the latter classifies the former and is therefore metacummunication." The content aspect simply transmits the message (or data), while the relationship aspect shows how the message is to be understood (p. 54).

His third axiom is: "The nature of a relationship is contingent upon the punctuation of the communicational sequences between the communicants" (p. 59). It is not a question of whether this punctuation is good or bad but simply that it organizes behavioral events (p. 56).

His fourth axiom is: "Human beings communicate both digitally and analogically. Digital language has a highly complex and powerful logical syntax but lacks inadequate semantics in the field of relationship, while analogic language possesses the semantics but has no adequate syntax for the unambiguous definition of the nature of relationships" (pp. 66–67). Human beings alone have at their disposal both analogic and digital modes of communication, analogic language signifying more archaic forms such as gesturing or tone of speech, and digital language signifying, for example, abstractions in language, or as Bateson puts it: "There is nothing particularly five-like about the number 'five'; there is nothing particularly table-like in the word 'table' " (Watzlawick, Beaver, & Jackson, 1967, p. 62).

His fifth axiom is: "All communicational interchanges are either symmetrical or complementary, depending on whether they are based on equality or difference" (p. 70). These axioms (which according to Watzlawick are only tentatively formulated) provide us with a well-structured instrument with which to observe interaction before becoming ensnared in interpretations, which make purpose-oriented interaction more difficult. Behavior, here, is not coupled as a stimulus/response pattern; nor is it related to Parson's notion of roles. I would suggest that in cases of interference in interaction one should look at the communication structures as drawn up by Watzlawick instead of resorting to the concept of stress, which King has built into her theory. It must be borne in mind that messages are not limited to the verbal (digital) plane, and that most frequently it is nonverbal messages in particular that make up the more direct plane that determines a relationship.

I would like once more to go into the reasons why I prefer an approach to interaction based on communication theory for nursing. In my view the psychodynamic approach does not make full use of the knowledge secured by the neurosciences. Taking over a specific role (as mother, daughter, teacher, etc.) as a surface of projection or transference may have its attraction for the patient and has undoubtedly proved effective in psychotherapeutic practice (for example, as suggested by Peplau, 1962); however, in a context of bioscience-oriented psychiatry or somatics clashes arise drawing nurses into interaction with neighboring professional groups in which there is a potential for conflict. They thus use up time and energy that would be better spent on interaction with the patient. This is not meant as a criticism of methods but as an appeal to examine whether theoretical approaches can be coupled with their respective practice. With regard to the humanistic approach, I have already stated my view above that it may be used to form a personal inner attitude but not misused as a moral stick to be wielded every day in the theory and practice of nursing. The world has enough ills to recover from without adding nursing to them. May I be allowed to observe that, as far as nursing's involvement and efficacy in the maturing and development of fellow humans is concerned, nurses have just as little cause for immodesty as other professional groups. Thus, the more sober the view of communication structures is regarding patients, their relatives, nursing's own, and other professions as well as the conditions under which things are organized, the more realistic the prospects are of being able to work effectively with all the valuable approaches that have been formulated in recent years.

PAIN AS A SYMBOL IN INTERACTION: A CASE TAKEN FROM TEACHING

Nurses are not entitled, in my view, to pass moral judgments about patterns of interaction in other systems before they have started to take a look at those operating within their own professional group. For this reason I would like to present an example from teaching practice at a nurses' training college that I have continued to study for some time now, partly in discussions with patients and medical staff.

I must firstly give a brief account of the circumstances. A class of 16 trainee nurses were presenting the results of the three working groups they had formed the previous day to draw up summaries of the theories put forward by Henderson, Peplau, and Orem. They had also been asked to express their own views on the particular theory they had been given to summarize. Two of the groups had little difficulty in accomplishing their task, but because the group working with Henderson's theory seemed to be having problems I worked predominantly with them. We became involved in a discussion about needs. One student offered the example of "imaginary headaches," to which another student added: "And once they've got one, they never leave off." After a while they succeeded in eliminating value judgments from their remarks and concentrated on seeking the needs of their patient without asking the doctor straight away to prescribe aspirin as they had intended to do in the beginning. Work on this question had taken quite a long time, and for me it represented a crucial part of this group's results. The following day the group presented Henderson's theory to the others; they were well prepared, with typed, very legible transparencies. They expressed themselves with great clarity—but they did not say a word about the case we had spent so much time and effort on the day before. The other groups performed equally well, articulating their ideas clearly, and presenting and explaining the concepts underlying the theories with apparent ease. What more could a teacher wish for, one might think. If only everything hadn't gone so quickly and smoothly. The content aspect was dealt with without a hitch; the relationship aspect likewise—even though it was only the second time in the group. But there was lively participation all round, no leaning back, students smiling, and no private conversations between neighbors, which didn't end promptly in the interest of the group. In fact, everything was fine—until I inquired about the case the Henderson group had worked on for so long the day before. "Which case? Oh, that one! We'd forgotten about that." I asked the students to look at the example of the headache once more from the point of view of the different theoretical approaches. Things started to become more arduous. Perhaps it wasn't a class that enjoyed theory after all. Was I asking too much of them? Or too little? Again contributions were to be heard like: "And once they think they've got a pain, many of them just never leave off," "Really, all they want is a bit of attention," and "Many of them aren't really in pain at all."

I told the students to examine the semantics and pragmatics of the symbol word pain. On account of the statements they had just uttered, I wrote on the left side of the blackboard the heading "Pain as a lie." Participation was lively and the case—right down to the patient's hyperventilation tetany, panic among the nurses, and a delegation sent to the doctor all because of a situation arising from the interaction between patient and nurse—was duly constructed and its structure analyzed. Cases were recounted from nursing practice; all the students joined in, and there was much laughter. We then went over to the right side of the board: "Pain as a symbol." Of what? The answers came hesitantly: "Of mental pain. Loneliness. Sorrow. Fear. Physical pain." Five earnest meanings of the symbol word pain. The class was quiet, the discussion laborious—a far cry from the other side of the board. I asked the students what the matter was; why there was suddenly no more participation. Was my question too difficult, or too easy? No, came the answer, there was nothing wrong. It was just that they had done something similar in the psychology class the day before. And, anyway, did one need to be so pedantic about certain words? Wasn't it clear enough what they meant. I shouldn't take it personally. Everything was okay, but enough was enough. I pointed to the board and simply asked whether there was a proper balance between the left and right sides: between the outcome of the discussion that pain was evaluated—provocatively expressed—as a lie and the outcome of the discussion in which it was a question of earnestly diagnosing a patient's needs. That they had no difficulty from the point of view of theory was something that I had already realized from their lively contributions. So where was the problem? With the chalk I drew a line down the middle of the blackboard, thus visually separating both sides. Spontaneously, a student answered, agitated: "I'm quite aware that we ought to go on from here. On the ward we mostly only take the one side into account so that we don't have to spend so much time on the patients. But I've got such a guilty conscience about it that I'd rather not go any deeper into it. . . . "

I will end my account of this example of teaching practice here, just as I ended my lecture on nursing theory at this point to give the students an opportunity to express their views. Every teacher at a nursing college knows how this story goes on ("Damn theory . . . damn practice"), but all will draw their own conclusions about how to deal with it.

It is easy, here, either to arrive at a moral assessment of the situation or to take a resigned attitude toward it. Or we might even hazard a psychological interpretation of the group's resistance. Alternatively, however, we can also follow the thread of the interaction by carrying out a continuous analysis of the communication. In this case the students themselves have already provided the result. No moral appeal was needed but, at the same time, no solution would have been possible if the communication had continued on the content plane. The student's naive underestimation of the complexity of interaction had already come to light by merely looking at the simple notion of pain. Here, we must achieve an awareness for the problems involved. It cannot be emphasized enough how important it is to develop communicative competence and a clinical ability to empathize that go beyond ordinary everyday understanding. Nurses have brought into existence the myth (probably nurtured from the myth of women's powers of feeling and understanding) that they possess a greater capacity for empathy than other professional groups. As a number of studies have demonstrated (Hunstein et al., 1997; Walter, 1996), this claim must unfortunately be contradicted. On the contrary, because of insufficient communicative competence (there is no lack of feeling but these feelings are vague), nurses are hardly in a position to interact adequately in encounters with all the different persons and groups who populate the health system. This leads to grave errors in assessing situations in the nursing process. It is no comfort to think that things are not much better in the medical profession.

INTERACTION IN NURSING: FURTHER REFLECTIONS

Now that I have presented interaction as a concept within a number of theoretical models and have attempted to illustrate the problems involved by taking an example from teaching, I would like to offer a few further reflections on interaction in nursing practice.

In agreement with Watzlawick, I assume first that interaction is a sequence of reciprocal messages between two or more persons. These messages are only partially of a verbal nature. They can also be understood in the tone of voice with its modulations; shades of color; as well as changes; different degrees of touch; and smells that permeate the air; secretions such as sweat, sputum, vomit, urine, feces, pus, blood, semen, menstrual blood, tears, which themselves are also connected with shades of color, smells, or noises. These elements of interaction are enumerated here for the sole reason that they are not mentioned by any of the interaction theorists except Goffman (1967, p. 80). He asserts that nurses who keep their distance from a patient out of consideration for the situation are likely to have a different facial expression from nurses who avoid patients because they smell or are incontinent. In his book he describes a number of situations that put the behavior of nursing staff in the context of social rituals, thus providing valuable stimuli for communication analyses.

In the great majority of books the interactants, although perhaps not able to express themselves with adequate coherence because of their mental state, are nevertheless physically healthy and clean human beings—even if they may sound rather lifeless from the authors' descriptions. But even in publications of Gestalt psychology, in which persons are at least allowed to breathe and move, there are no patients with ozena or other foul-smelling ailments among the case illustrations. No great studies are necessary to demonstrate that such factors play a decisive role in influencing interaction. What we must do, however, is examine the ways in which these factors affect behavior because it is quite clear that in their dealings with each other nurses and patients/clients are continuously involved with all of their senses. It will thus no longer suffice in our investigation of interaction to confine ourselves to the field of verbal and nonverbal communication as it has been interpreted up to present (i.e., as demeanor, gestures, or signs). We need to carry out studies that, beyond a phenomenology of disgust, examine its effects on communication in a pragmatic way. Real-life communication is a highly complex system that each individual perceives and directs selectively for his or her own ends. Interaction is also influenced by such elements of communication as colors (Wied, 1998), room furnishings and design, acoustics, or technical equipment. A dyadic view of the interaction between nurse and patient is no longer commensurate with today's advances in the communication sciences. How an individual or the system nursing as a professional group selects its perceptions depends to a considerable extent, furthermore, on training and attitudes. Thus, in my view, it is no longer possible to view the notion of relationship as merely the relationship between two persons; it must now be defined as the relationship between the messages of two or more persons. This brings about a shift of perspective that has its effects on the organization of practice. As far as the notions of interaction and communication are concerned, the division between psychiatric and somatic nursing with their emphases on the mental and physical aspects of care, respectively, becomes superfluous if we make use of an approach based on a systemic communications theory that is contextually linked with nursing and caring.

REFERENCES

Canetti, E. (1976). *Die Provinz des Menschen.* Hamburg, Germany: Fischer. (Quoted passage translated by G. Nixon.)

Canetti, E. (1978). *The human province* (J. Neugroschel, Trans.). New York: Farrar, Strauss, Giroux.

Der Duden (1982). *Das Fremdwörterbuch.* Vol. 6. Mannheim, Germany: Duden.

Fawcett, J. (1993). *Analysis and evaluation of nursing theories.* Philadelphia: Davis.

Fawcett, J. (1995). *Analysis and evaluation of conceptual models of nursing* (3rd ed.). Philadelphia: Davis.

Fawcett, J. (1996). *Pflegemodelle im Überblick.* Bern, Germany: Huber.

Fuchs-Heinritz, W. (Ed.). (1994). *Lexikon der Soziologie.* Opladen, Germany: Westdeutscher Verlag.

Goffman, I. (1967). *Interaction ritual: Essays in face-to-face behavior.* Chicago: Aldine.

Guttman, P. (1990). In W. Tschacher (Ed.), *Interaktion in selbstorganisierten Systemen* (p. 148). Heidelberg, Germany: Asanger

Hunstein, D., Dreut, M., Eckert, S., et al. (1997). Wie erlehen patienten aus anderen kulturen das deutsche gesundheitswesen? (How do patients from other cultures experience the German health system?) *Pflege.* Bern, Germany: Huber.

King, I. M. (1981). *A theory for nursing: Systems, concepts, process.* Albany, NY: Delmar.

Luhmann, N. (1996). *Soziale Systeme.* Frankfurt, Germany: Suhrkamp.

Mead, G. H. (1934). *Mind, self, and society from the stand-point of a social behaviorist.* Chicago: University of Chicago Press.

Meleis, A. (1991). *Theoretical nursing: Development and progress* (2nd ed.). Philadelphia: Lippincott.

Parsons, T. (1949). *The structure of social action.* Glencoe, IL: The Free Press.

Paterson, J. G., & Zderad, L. T. (1970/1971). All together through complementary syntheses. *Image, 4,* 13–16.

Paterson, J. G., & Zderad, L. T. (1988). *Humanistic nursing.* New York: National League for Nursing.

Peplau, H. E. (1962). *Interpersonal relations in nursing.* New York: Putnam.

Tschacher, W. (1990). *Interaktion in selbstorganisierten Systemen.* Heidelberg, Germany: Asanger. (Quoted passage translated by G. Nixon.)

Walter, A. (1996). *A qualitative study of values as expressed by young people in training.* Berlin, Germany: Humboldt University.

Watzlawick, P., Beaver, J. H., & Jackson, D. D. (1967). *Pragmatics of human communication: A study of interactional patterns, pathologies, and paradoxes.* New York: Norton.

Watzlawick, P., Beaver, J. H., & Jackson, D. D. (1996). *Menschliche Kommunikation.* (A German translation). Bern, Germany: Huber.

Wied, S. (1998). *Das phänomen der farbe und ihrer wahrnehmung (The phenomenon of color and its perception).* Unpublished doctoral dissertation, Humboldt University, Berlin.

Wittgenstein, L. (1977). *Tractatus Logico-Philosophicus*, D. F. Pears & B. F. McGuinness, trans. London: Routledge & Kegan Paul. (Original work published in 1921.)

Wörterbuch der Psychiatrie und medizinischen Psychologie (Dictionary of psychiatry and medical psychology). (1977). München, Germany: Urban und Schwartzenberg.

Zderad, L. (1969). Empathic nursing. *Nursing Clinics of North America, 4,* 655–662.

6

The Concept of Culture and Transculturality*

Charlotte Uzarewicz

Introducing the notion of *culture* into nursing and nursing science is both meaningful and necessary to inquire into and learn to understand dimensions of human action and behavior in nursing other than those that have hitherto been discussed and investigated. This chapter aims to clarify the semantics of culture as used in nursing and health care, pointing out ideological pitfalls inherent in the meanings of culture used in philosophy and commonsensically. There are two major tendencies in the use of culture: one that is based on epistemological treatment and the other a normative usage as in racism. To be able to disengage these two tendencies, the precise use of language is essential when dealing with culture. In the following, culture is revealed to be a purely notional construct that has no concrete equivalent in empirical reality: culture and cultures as entities do not exist. The cultural is therefore discussed as a basic phenomenological structure, as the basis of the social, which cuts across the social strata of society and the boundaries of the national state. Our actions and our behavior are, of course, to be seen against a cultural background; however, the assertion that a Turk or a German behaves in a certain way or that something is typically German or typically American is false. If such assertions are not to be understood as prejudices or stereotypes, then one can speak merely of ideal types, modal types, or statistical averages.

Because the problems arising from the issue of culture are related to otherness, to the alien, these are given special consideration. The smaller the world becomes, the greater the role that is played by the cultural, particularly in situations marked by existential crisis such as illness and

*Translated from German by Gerald Nixon.

distress, with which nurses and care givers are frequently confronted. Thus, the example of the culture-bound syndrome is used to illustrate the relevance of the cultural to nursing.

CULTURE

In a general social scientific sense the concept of culture is divided into three domains: (1) artifacts (i.e., architecture, clothing, music, language, etc.); (2) categories (such as time and space); and, (3) human relationships (both intracultural and intercultural). In cultural research the attempt is made to identify and study qualitatively the areas of interconnection and exchange between these three domains. In the following analysis the various definitions of culture—be they psychological/cognitive, materialistic, and so forth—are given no consideration.[1] Here, culture means in the broadest sense the social sediment (the basis) in which human actions and behavior take place. Moreover (and this must be made clear from the very beginning) because the cultural undergoes constant change historically, it is something fundamentally dynamic. By contrast, culture in its substantivized form always appears to be a (closed) entity and suggests substance. Culture as a monolithic concept attempts to conceal all heterogeneity and differentiation under the ideological mantle of unity. Subsequently, out of this unity springs the demand for a cultural identity as an important and essential factor for every human being. That our use of the term culture is just as difficult from an epistemological point of view as it is generally valid from a normative point of view lies in the fact that the characterizations of its contents are never unequivocally establishable. "On account of their symbolic character every culture and every element of culture can have more than one interpretation and are susceptible to shifts of meaning,compression, etc. . . . Culture is thus the field of battle for meanings, for cultural hegemony . . . , particularly in times of social upheaval. . . . " (Auernheimer, 1989, pp. 386–387). Geiger (1988) reveals the extent to which scientific analyses on the subject of culture can be categorized as belonging to the politically right or the politically left spectrum of argumentation—whereby neither orientation recognizes the crux of the problem arising from the concept of culture: (a) a normatively applied concept of culture possesses its own dialectic moment, which can be expressed as the contradiction between the "right to be equal and . . . the right to be different" (Geiger, 1998, p. 89); and (b) everyone has the right to one's own individual uniqueness and cultural particularity, while at the same time all human beings are equal.

A normatively applied concept of culture serves as a guide to self-orientation: the question "Where do I belong?" can be answered with reference to a particular cultural identity, whatever form this may take. The self-assurance in one's behavior toward others and the other that purportedly results from this sense of belonging is based on the axiom that one is rooted in a culture (implied are biological roots; see below). Such norm-oriented behavior bears witness to normality, but at the same time it is also evidence of deviance in cases in which the cultural markers, or imprints, are disdained. To this extent the concept of culture creates a basis for discriminatory action and behavior. The normative pitfall is to be seen in the ideologizing of cultural patterns of behavior: personal habits as well as likes and dislikes are taken to be typical of a culture. People born by pure chance in a certain country are made members of a culture, a people, or a nation. Thus, culture is always a differentiating term (whether in the singular or plural). Within the society of a nation state it can have a stratifying effect and form hierarchies: (high) culture is hegemonistic because its codes and norms acquire universal validity in social discourses. Having such a dominant position, it can act against the subcultures existing in the same society. Between the societies of two nation states culture—as national culture—becomes a factor of distinction.

In summary, it can be said that the issue of culture mainly arises when dealing with phenomena of the other, the others, or the alien. Today, in scientific as well as in political or everyday discussions, the semantic field of the normative concept of culture has been enriched by the terms otherness, nationality, and ethnos/ethnicity. As a substantivized term it serves to determine the inclusion or exclusion of individuals or groups. In its adjectival use, too, enhanced by various prefixes, it serves primarily to draw boundaries and distinguish otherness, as in multicultural society, intercultural dialogue, transcultural nursing. For this reason it is worthwhile to seek clarification of these implications on an epistemological plane.

ETHNOS, RACE, AND CULTURE

If one takes a closer look at the semantic field of the cultural, terms denoting ethnicity, nationality, and otherness almost automatically emerge from the shadow of culture. What these terms have in common is "that they not only express the way people see themselves in certain historical situations but also provide criteria, mechanisms and practices of inclusion and exclusion" (Müller, 1993, p. 52). In this process, there has been a strange mixing of the connotations of these terms. Ethnos, an administrative concept familiar in antiquity, was first defined in ethnology as a process (Shirokogoroff, 1923). Later, the term lost its dynamic aspect and denoted a specific group situated, according to quantity and quality, somewhere between family, clan, and nation state (Ganzer, 1990, p. 14). Haller uses the criteria of "a collective name; a common mythical origin; a common history; a specific common culture; association with a specific territory; a sense of belonging or solidarity" (Haller, 1993, p. 33) to define ethnos, while other definitions include the aspect of "biological unity," "characterized by passing on the genotype endogamously" (Giordano, 1981, p. 181). The fact that such broadly formulated definitions can be filled with all manners of contents explains why the term appears equally acceptable from the outer as well as from the inner perspective. Empirical reality is quite different, however: ethnic groups as discrete, homogeneous units do not exist. On the contrary, there is a continuous process of assimilation, adaptation through immigration and emigration, and adoption of individuals or whole groups as well as the integration of cultural artifacts or behavior through trade and other forms of contact (Mühlmann, 1985, pp. 10ff). Attributes or natural qualities simply cannot be ascribed to all or even the majority of the individuals regarded as belonging to an ethnic group; neither, as a rule, is there a single language spoken by the whole group; nor a national territory (i.e., an area exclusively and inclusively settled); nor values, norms, rules, and laws that are acknowledged by all. And biological features are even less helpful in the classification of ethnic groups. Science has thus constructed a term to interpret reality; consequently, what is said about actual ethnic groups acquires universal validity.

Of significance in these definitions for our context is the amalgamation of cultural, historical, religious, and naturalistic aspects. The paradigm of descent—whether understood in terms of mythology or biology—is to be found in all terms in which a common origin, common roots, or a common basis is written into the definition as a group's lowest common denominator. When descent is viewed biologically, one arrives at the concept of race,[2] which itself contains two different yet related elements: the explanation of race makes reference to nature, out of which specific social forms and a capacity to act are then derived (Dittrich & Radtke, 1990, p. 18). How, then, are nature and culture (as social forms) related in the notional constructs—how are they interconnected? Classical physical anthropology in Germany[3] studied individual bodies (e.g., skull shapes or bone length) to establish a typology. Human beings were categorized by means of their anatomy. Today's gene analysis technology has radicalized this inductive, empirical method. As a result, however, universally valid precepts regarding human typology are no longer possible (Cavalli-Sforza and Cavalli-Sforza, 1994). Race as a collective concept—a category—has become obsolete. Its place has been taken by other collective concepts, such as culture[4] or ethnos.[5] The attempt is no longer made, inductively, to stand these on an empirical basis; on the contrary, assertions are deduced from them.[6] What is qualitatively new about this culturalist change of course is the disappearance of the individual (body). Inferences are no longer made about character from anatomy or biology; conversely, "the cultural, as a collective attribute of the people, determines the appearance and character of the individual—and unalterably so" (Uzarewicz & Uzarewicz, 1998, p. 146). This substitution of the sociocultural for the biological determination of the individual is basically an attempt to achieve a "naturalization of social relationships" (Müller, 1993, p. 56). Biology is no longer individualist, as it was in craniometry and physical anthropology, but is used in a collectivist way in concepts of common origin or a genetic pool. Whereas in the former method it was still possible to see individual differences, these no longer play any role in the latter approach. In a concept of ethnos bound with ancestry, language, way of life, culture, tradition, and a system of values the individual is eliminated. The group, mass, or monad is basically considered to be of a different kind and is established as the cultural constant, which acquires validity as the basis of ethnic or cultural identity. Race and ethnos are thus mere constructs of the natural and social sciences and have no natural equivalent in reality. Problems arise in such collective concepts whenever they are to be measured by the yardstick of empirical reality. What is everyday life like in a large city with neighbors from all over the world? Classifying culture as Turkish, German, or Greek negates the process of continuous cultural exchange—and change—that exists in the real world. Ideological assumptions are hypostatized and become absolute values; this sells well in political discourse as the conservation of the cultural legacy, cultural identity, and a multicultural society—understood as various groups of people living side by side. However, such a normative drive brings with it the threat of the individual or the group being uprooted, the loss of a sense of purpose, and disorientation in the life of these individuals when their own cultural roots are held in low esteem. Thus, it is obvious that both ethnos and culture can be used as catchwords of political struggle.

> It appears that terms like 'racial' or 'ethnic', which are widely used in this connection not only by sociology but also by the broad mass of people, are symptoms of an ideological defense. Using them diverts attention toward

> minor aspects of this figuration (e.g., differences in skin color) and away from the crucial aspect (differences in power). (Elias & Scotson, 1993, p. 27)[7]

By adhering to ancestry and origin, culturalist concepts remain naturalistic. When cultural and ethnic identity are brought up in modern discourse, the biological aspect no longer needs to be explicitly named; the secret knowledge of it is tantamount to a taboo. The new categories can be employed in the social and cultural sciences in all manners of ways as dimensions of a theory of action or as a basic model of society. It is not coincidental that the axioms of biological and cultural roots are no longer distinguished. A tautological circle thus arises in which whatever was created first can be verified by the same means.

PROBLEMS OF OTHERNESS[8]

Otherness is an elementary and existential experience. No one can see what is going on in another person's mind—regardless of the gender, political system, nationality, ethnic group, or culture ascribed to that person. One has always to rely on the assumption and the hope that one is understood by the others. People living in modern societies are confronted in real life with culturally defined strangers[9] to a far greater degree than those of other much more self-contained societies of the past. Eifler and Saame even talk of the "everyday experience of 'other-ness' and the feeling of alienation in a mass industrial and high technology society" (1991, p. 12). The traditional authorities and institutions (e.g., religion) that used to guarantee security and certainty are slowly disintegrating and becoming obsolete. What consequences does this have for individual action and behavior? On the epistemological plane otherness is a paradoxical term because otherness cannot be put into words; on the other hand, this is exactly what the term implies: a description of what cannot be described. This paradox contains an aspect that is of considerable importance for the whole issue: the aspect of power. Only if otherness as such can be categorized is it possible to find a corresponding mode of behavior. If it is neither recognizable nor perceptible, it is not only "not other" but also cognitively nonexistent. Denoting a thing or a person by the term *other* is the first step toward understanding, toward nostrification. Putting something into words, finding a term for something, means making it more controllable, reducing its otherness. The original fear of being subject to the power of something other, something alien, is reversed; the more one knows about this something, the more power one gains over it.[10] The result of this, however, is that the term becomes a normative problem, for human existence is nothing other than a permanent process of practical nostrification. Gehlen notes:

> Human beings are thus organically "deficient creatures" (Herder). They would be unable to survive in any natural environment and so they must first create a second nature, an artificial made-to-measure substitute world suited to their inadequate organic apparatus. And this they do wherever they are encountered. They live, so to speak, in an artificially detoxicated world, convenient and specially modified to suit their life-style. . . . (Gehlen, 1961, p. 48)

The whole history of humankind can be interpreted as a (theoretical) process of getting rid of the other (nostrification) (Bude, 1994; Stagl, 1981). Chaos is replaced by order, nature by culture, the other (depending on the mode of interpretation) by the known, the recognized, the new or one's own—and cognitively acquired. It is from this vital necessity that spring the difficulties and the problems that people have with the alien. Whatever resists stereotyping and classification or cannot be subsumed remains diffuse, amorphous, unresolved. As can easily be seen, the problem does not have its source primarily in the thing, in otherness, but in perception itself.[11] As long as ambiguity and ambivalence characterize otherness, it represents a threat to the binary logic of occidental conceptions of order (Baumann, 1992). It is for this reason that most people react first and foremost with suspicion, fear, and resistance. Seeing the other as something desirable or exotic takes only second place. And in accordance with the logic of differentiation and identity described above, there are clear strategies of action for dealing with the problem of the other or others and for guaranteeing one's own supposed safety: whatever is not me must be neutralized; either it becomes (or is made) like me, adapted to me, or it is subjected to strict control—in the most intractable of cases it is eliminated. Everything must be comprehensible and governable, and thus in (best) order—this is the program of the modern integration.

The more natural the cultural categories appear, the easier it is to achieve success in this. By thinking of other (alien) people in natural categories, it is easier to subsume them under this power. It is ultimately racist or quite general naturalistic cultural stereotypes that ascribe special attributes to those who are very different. In this way groups can be divided into one's own and other, and social, political, and economic hierarchies can be constructed. In case of doubt, anyone or anything that does not correspond to notions of what is common to one's own group can be considered alien. Alien and one's own are not anthropological or ontological categories in themselves; they are social constructs.[12] In modern history the application to the human sphere of the difference between culture and nature has undergone a modification in the terms used. In the past it was customary to speak—unequivocally and unashamedly—of cultured, civilized peoples (one's own) and natural, primitive peoples (aliens, in foreign lands).[13] Through the naturalizing of culture this crude categorization has been superseded by a more subtle mechanism of differentiation. The other culture (there is no longer any need to speak of nature) is per se quite different from one's own, and both are regarded as distinct and separate worlds. Attached to this other world, however, is an aura of diffuseness, indeterminacy, betweenness.[14]

This alien, as a potential or actual migrant between the two worlds, has the (seeming) advantage over the indigenous group that he can revoke his choice of domicile and return to where he came from. The mere opportunity of being able to choose is regarded as a provocation of ordinary everyday understanding. Belonging neither to the one nor the other, he negates all collective identity. This is clearly seen in the modern terminology, in which new words are constantly being thought up for such aliens: migrants, asylum-seekers, refugees, and so forth are a threat to one's own collective identity but, at the same time, such an identity is denied them. Hence, they are branded aliens. In their cultural ghetto the sanctuary that they are granted for their identity is for the most part only of a folkloristic nature.

Even though the aliens scarcely have a chance of being accepted, they must constantly prove their worth by not only expressing verbally but also showing in their actions and behavior a more than sufficient degree of identity with their host society and its values and norms—more, in fact, than anything that is required from a member of that society: "with twice as much devotion, diligence and dogged self-denial" (Horkheimer & Adorno, 1986, p. 183). The aliens must correspond as perfectly as possible to the image that the reference group has of itself. Nevertheless, there is no escape from the ambivalence of their status because, at least once, they have betrayed their roots in the eyes of all others by leaving their homeland. For the rest of their lives they are predestined—as newcomers—to be scapegoats, and it is possible that this will be true of their children and their children's children, too. On the other hand, through this overidentification with the host society they make themselves all the more suspicious, especially as its members can hardly find it agreeable to be constantly faced with their own self-image—and thus their own shortcomings—even if aliens succeed in conforming to this image at least partially. The aliens remain, for good or for ill, at the mercy of the capricious benevolence of their environment because, from a legal point of view, too, they are in an inferior and more vulnerable position, should they belong to a different nationality.[15]

CONCEPTUALIZING TRANSCULTURALITY FOR NURSING SCIENCE

The above observations on culture and otherness were intended to make clear that because of the diffuse and contradictory character of their contents a substantivized use of the terms is in no way suited to making unequivocal assertions and even less as a guide for taking action. They may well possess considerable power in social politics; in the context of the social sciences, however, they are highly complicated and controversial. A substantivized and substantialist form of the term culture makes no sense from an epistemological standpoint; in normative terms—as has been demonstrated above—it is highly explosive in a sociopolitical framework. Nevertheless, the existence of cultural differences cannot be denied (even though they must not be hypostasized into cultures). They relate to both the social interaction between nurses and patients as well as to institutions: the structures of care provision in a society, their accessibility for those who need them, levels of health, care for the elderly, and so forth. In both cases cultural symbols or processes, as "life's medium, pure and simple" (Lipp, 1979, p. 465) are the links between the social categories of society (*Gesellschaft*) and community (*Gemeinschaft*): they are the basis of all social interaction and integral components of every institution. For nursing and caring the cultural is of special significance because if people are sensitive in dealing with it, it opens up new paths of access to human behavior, especially in illnesses and situations of distress that cannot be adequately confronted from a medical, psychological, or sociological perspective.[16] The example of the culture-bound syndrome (CBS) may be used to illustrate the extent to which an understanding of the cultural is meaningful. The CBS, which has succeeded the concept of folk-illness, is a notion derived from Western biomedicine. It was used first to denote those disorders that could not be identified and classified by the nosological system of orthodox medicine. What is notable is the fact that in the descriptions of symptoms behavioral and awareness disorders predominated, while somatic ailments tended to play a minor role. Allopathic medicine had neither understanding for nor competence to deal with such phenomena.

The designation culture-bound syndrome inevitably led to the assumption that there were also culture-free sicknesses, which orthodox medicine would regard as diseases proper. Such a eurocentric perspective makes it possible to regard other (alien), not immediately comprehensible phenomena as culture-bound, thus creating a category that covers our own lack of understanding and ability to deal with them. We know today that every medical system is embedded in its specific sociocultural and historic context—and this is true of orthodox medicine, too. The significance of CBS would be easier to grasp if its name was culture-specific syndrome: this would include the types of disorder "which cannot be understood if deprived of their cultural or subcultural contexts, whereby their etiology is summed up and symbolized by key fields of meaning and behavioral norms of this society" (Greifeld, 1995, p. 24). For example, in our own cultural context the CBS complex includes such disorders as the premenstrual syndrome, bulimia, adiposity, and anorexia nervosa; in other cultural contexts these sicknesses are either not considered to be pathological or do not exist. The culture-specific features of patterns and types of illness are based on the conceptualization of the body or embodiment in a given society, which, as such, also reflect the social system of that society. M. Mauss speaks of body techniques in this connection, meaning, "the way people of different societies use their bodies according to tradition" (Mauss, 1978, p. 106). The "body as a social construction . . . governs the way in which the body is perceived as a physical construction" (Douglas, 1974, p. 99). Douglas (1974, p. 106) regards the body as a reflection of the society it exists in; according to her there is nothing natural about it, for example the different ways of walking, crouching, swimming, carrying objects on the head, and so forth.

Such cultural differences in conceptions of the body or embodiment, which are also related to those of spirit and soul(s), gain special significance when, in an age in which the world is becoming smaller, societies are becoming polycultural. For example, the orifices of the body (eyes, nose, mouth, etc.) are often thought of as being doors—points of entry for invading good or evil spirits. Consequently, they demand special attention. What happens to and what takes place in a patient's perceptions of one's own body when an endoscope is introduced into the stomach via the nose or an injection is given, causing direct contact with the interior of the body? This means that strangers have direct access to not only one's body but also inside the body, the whole personality. What are the implications of this for the way one feels about recovering one's health? From the point of view of orthodox medicine such a measure may be considered a vital necessity; for the patient it may be experienced as an attempt on one's own life. Further, in many societies the blood is regarded as the seat of life or of the life spirits. What significance does this have, then, when a blood sample is taken for routine testing? It may result in a gradual but progressive weakening of the body because in a different cultural awareness the life spirits are being drawn out of the body with the blood. When talking to the patient, taking into account the patient's specific background can reduce the patient's fears; it is conceivable that, on the treatment side, medical staff recognize that so-called routine tests are superfluous, and that blood samples may be dispensed with—or that the patient comes to acknowledge the necessity of the blood tests. A blood transfusion can cause similar problems, allowing alien spirits to invade the body, thus changing the person/personality in a way that is impossible for the individual to judge. Loss of identity and even mental disorders may be the result. For transcultural nursing this means, first, that an extensive store of knowledge is necessary (and accessible) to which nurses can refer; second, it means that what is needed is a trained eye, an analytic mind, the ability to differentiate, imagination, and above all empathy to be able, in case of doubt, to depart from the precepts of one's own medical system (or one's own system of interpretation) and go in search of others. Things can often be settled by talking to patients tactfully if they are well enough to respond. Here, communicative competence is required that goes beyond the scope of therapeutic conversations.

The concept of transculturality can be helpful in this context.[17] It places emphasis on phenomena as dynamic processes, thus corresponding more closely to today's empirical reality of cultural change, assimilation, adaptation, and migration than the notion of interculturality. Inter, meaning between, ultimately aims at upholding the borders that become permeable when contact takes place, for example as cultural comparisons. Internationality, for instance, is a bilateral concept between France and Germany; the European Union and NATO, by contrast, are transnational. These structures constitute something completely new: they leave the old nations behind while absorbing their substance in a process of synthesis. Brink (1976, p. 1) points to the transcendent character of transcultural nursing: in a Hegelian sense borders are removed, revoked and crossed. The phenomenon of doctor shopping described in ethnomedical literature is to be understood in this very way. In emergencies—and illness represents an emergency—people seize every opportunity offered them to recover their health. Accordingly, paying a visit to a doctor trained in orthodox medicine and consulting an oracle is by no means a contradiction but merely an attempt to combine and take advantage of the possibilities that are known and available.

Not only do human beings have a common biological, anthropological basis; above all, they are also creatures given to both creating and interpreting symbols. From the perspective of cultural history the dialectics between the right to be the same and the right to be different is to be understood in this context. In Brink's definition, in which transcultural nursing is defined as "nursing that transcends cultural boundaries seeking to find the essence of nursing that applies in all cultural contexts" (Brink, 1976, p. 1) one must bear in mind that it is not only a question of the essence of nursing in itself, which is to be found in all cultural contexts. What matters even more is that human interaction with symbols—as a cultural, anthropological constant—is just as important as the basic biological structures. For human beings there is no other way of perceiving and appropriating the world than interpreting it. The doctor shopping referred to above contains intercultural aspects because the patient is aware of the cultural boundaries and crosses from one side to the other. Furthermore, a crossing of boundaries also takes place in a transcendent sense because the patient absorbs various methods and synthesizes them. The overall effect is that something new arises that ultimately leads to the recovery of the patient's health. From this point of view transcultural nursing can be understood as the knowledge of one's own cultural foundations, the knowledge of other cultural phenomena, and the synthesis of both in a particular context of human action. Since this context of action invariably occurs in the form of personal interaction, the aspect of interaction dynamics is also an integral part of the concept. Epistemologically, as well as in practice, the concept of transculturality makes more sense (than that of interculturality) because little account needs to be taken of what for the most part exists in academic brains: the boundaries between cultures.

NOTES

1. See the comprehensive and still relevant compilation of culture concepts and their meanings undertaken by Kroeber, A. L., and Kluckhohn, C. (1952).
2. On the term race and the concept of race, see also Allport (1971, p. 121).
3. By classical physical anthropology we mean the branch of anthropology whose proponents included Blumenbach, Agassiz, Camper, Carus, and Soemmering. Parallel to this was a branch that proceeded in a more deductive fashion, taking the results of the aforementioned as their starting point and mixing them with social Darwinist approaches. Among the latter were Gobineau, Chamberlain, and so forth.

4. Cf. Konrad Lorenz, who in his works after 1945 replaced the notion of race by the notion of culture.
5. Cf. Stuart Hall (1980).
6. This is illustrated by Max Weber (1980, p. 528), using the collective concept of nation. He notes that as long as such concepts are not empirically validated they are of purely heuristic value.
7. A further crucial aspect, closely linked to power, is the economy. Capital has always been international and has never paid any heed to cultural borders.
8. The following observations are based on Uzarewicz & Uzarewicz (1998, pp. 236ff).
9. Strictly speaking, this statement is tautologous. The social form of a society is defined by the fact it is made up of strangers; a community does not know strangers—it only knows others.
10. This is why colonialism was a logical consequence of the Enlightenment.
11. On the various patterns of interpretation of the alien, see Mersch (1997, pp. 27ff), Schäffter (1991, p. 14), Ohle (1978, pp. 62–63), Oevermann (1983, p. 284), Weinrich (1985, pp. 24ff), and Guttandin (1993, pp. 458ff).
12. Social constructs are interiorized through processes of socialization or enculturation. Even what is one's own has to be learned.
13. This is more obvious in the German, which distinguished between *Kulturvölker* and *Naturvölker.*
14. To this realm of darkness (shadiness, quagmire, morass, wretchedness) belong the (criminal) underworld, the (archaic) world before, and the (primitive) world behind. Their distinguishing features are chaos, disorder, mystery, darkness, incomprehensibility, irrationality, sensuousness (music, dance, sexuality, intoxication, ecstasy), impurity, mire, acting on instinct, restlessness (migrants, nomads); their media are myths, sagas, fairy tales, stories and rumors with their fabulous creatures (fairies, hobgoblins, ghosts, demons, spirits, dervishes, sirens, creatures with dogs' heads, lotus-eaters)—but also women, Jews, children, gypsies, the insane, Blacks, Indians, savages, and primitive tribes (cf. Schütz, 1991, Vol. 2, p. 198).
15. The more corporate, government-led and self-contained a society is, the greater everyday xenophobia and its stereotyping seems to be. In the lament "I am denied what is entitled to me as a German," the state appears as the caring patriarch protecting his (own) family and children from misfortune. The belief that one is being neglected brings

forth feelings of jealousy towards the alien, who is thought to be stealing the favor of the fatherland.

16. The cultural as an epistemological concept reveals nothing about the consequences that arise for social action. On the contrary, consequences for action are left for all individuals to decide according to their senses of responsibility.
17. Madeleine Leininger applied the term transculturality to the context of nursing to describe her observations of nursing in New Guinea. Her belief that culture and nursing exert a mutual influence on one another has become a concept that is no longer disputed. It can thus be considered to be a very successful concept. However, one must not make the mistake of regarding the term as being irrevocably bound to the thoughts of its author. One can more readily grasp its significance and its theoretical as well as practical consequences from the nature of the word itself.

REFERENCES

Allport, G. W. (1971). *Die Natur des Vorurteils.* Köln, Germany: Kiepenheuer & Witsch.

Auernheimer, G. (1989). Kulturelle Identität—ein gegenaufklärerischer Mythos? *Das Argument, 175,* 381–394.

Baumann, Z. (1992). *Moderne und Ambivalenz. Das Ende der Eindeutigkeit.* Hamburg, Germany: Junius Verlag.

Brink, P. (1976). Introduction. In P. Brink (Ed.), *Transcultural nursing. A Book of Readings.* Englewood Cliffs, NJ: Prentice-Hall.

Bude, H. (1994). Das Latente und das Manifeste. Aporien einer "Hermeneutik des Verdachts." In D. Garz (Hg.), *Die Welt als Text* (pp. 114–124). Frankfurt, Germany: Suhrkamp.

Cavalli-Sforza, L., & Cavalli-Sforza, F. (1994). *Verschieden und doch gleich. Ein Genetiker entzieht dem Rassismus die Grundlagen.* München, Germany: Droemer Knaur.

Dittrich, E. J., & Radtke, F. (Hg.). (1990). *Ethnizität. Wissenschaft und Minderheiten.* Opladen, Germany: Westduetscher Verlag.

Douglas, M. (1974). *Ritual, Tabu und Körpersymbolik. Sozialanthropologische Studien in Industriegesellschaften und Stammeskulturen.* Frankfurt, Germany: Suhrkamp.

Eifler, G., & Saame, O. (Hg.) (1991). *Das Fremde. Aneignung und Ausgrenzung. Eine interdisziplinäre Erörterung.* Wien, Germany: Böhlau-Verlag.

Elias, N., & Scotson, J. L. (1993). *Etablierte und Außenseiter.* Frankfurt, Germany: Suhrkamp.

Ganzer, B. (1990). Zur Bestimmung des Begriffs der ethnischen Gruppe. *Sociologus, Heft, 1,* NF: 3–18.

Gehlen, A. (1961). *Anthropologische Forschung.* Hamburg, Germany: Rowohlt.

Geiger, K. F. (1998). Vorsicht: Kultur. Stichworte zu kommunizierendem Denken. *Das Argument, 224,* 81–90.

Giordano, C. (1981). Ethnizität: Soziale Bewegung oder Identitätsmanagement. *Schweizerische Zeitschrift für Soziologie, 7,* 179–198.

Greifeld, K. (1995). Einführung in die Medizinethnologie. In B. Pfleiderer, K. Greifeld, & W. Bichmann (Hg.), *Ritual und Heilung. Eine Einführung in die Ethnomedizin* (pp. 11–31). Berlin, Germany: Reimer Verlag.

Guttandin, F. (1993). Die Relevanz des hermeneutischen Verstehens für eine Soziologie des Fremden. In T. Jung, & S. Müller-Doohm (Hg.), *"Wirklichkeit" im Deutungsprozeß. Verstehen und Methoden in den Kultur- und Sozialwissenschaften* (pp. 458–481). Frankfurt, Germany: Suhrkamp.

Hall, S. (1980). Rasse—Klasse—Ideologie. *Das Argument.* Heft Nr. 122.

Haller, M. (1993). Klasse und Nation. Konkurrierende und komplementäre Grundlagen kollektiver Identität und kollektiven Handelns. *Soziale Welt, Heft, 1,* 30–51.

Horkheimer, M., & Adorno, T. W. (1986). *Dialektik der Aufklärung.* Frankfurt, Germany: Fischer. (Original work published 1947)

Kroeber, A. L., & Kluckhohn, C. (1952). *Culture. A critical review of concepts and definitions.* New York: University Press.

Lipp, W. (1979). Kulturtypen, kulturelle Symbole, Handlungswelt. *Kölner Zeitschrift für Soziologie und Sozialpsychologie, 31,* 450–484.

Mauss, M. (1978). *Soziologie und Anthropologie. Bd.2.* Frankfurt, Germany: Ullstein.

Mersch, D. (1997). Vom anderen Reden. Das Paradox der Alterität. In M. Brocker & H. H. Nau (Hg.), *Ethnozentrismus. Möchlichkeiten und Grenzen des interkulturellen Dialogs* (pp. 27–45). Darmstadt, Germany: Wissenschaftliche Buchgesellschaft.

Mühlmann, W. E. (1985). *Studien zur Ethnogenese. Abhandlungen der Rheinisch-Westfälischen Akademie der Wissenschaften. 72.Bd.* Opladen, Germany: Westdeutscher Verlag.

Müller, H. (1993). Rasse, Ethnos, Kultur und Nation. Eine Phänomenologie zentraler Begriffe im Diskurs um die Migrationsgesellschaft. In M. J. Gorzini & H. Müller (Hg.), *Handbuch zur interkulturellen Arbeit* (pp. 52–69). Mainz, Germany: Wissenschaftiche Buchgesellschaft Darmstadt.

Oevermann, U. (1983). Zur Sache. Die Bedeutung von Adornos methodologischem Selbstverständnis für die Begründung einer materialen soziologischen Strukturanalyse. In L. V. Friedeburg & J. Habermas (Hg.), *Adorno-Konferenz 1983* (pp. 234–289). Frankfurt, Germany: Suhrkamp.

Ohle, K. (1978). *Das Ich und das Andere. Grundzüge einer Soziologie des Fremden. Sozialwissenschaftliche Studien 15.* Stuttgart, Germany: Gustav Fischer Verlag.

Schäffter, O. (Hg.) (1991). *Das Fremde. Erfahrungsmöglichkeiten zwischen Faszination und Bedrohung.* Opladen, Germany: Nijhoff-Verlag.

Schütz, A. (1991). *Der sinnhafte Aufbau der sozialen Welt.* Frankfurt, Germany: Suhrkamp. (Original work published 1932.)

Shirokogoroff, S. M. (1923). *Ethnos. Allgemeine Prinzipien der Variationen von ethnographischen und ethnischen Phänomenen.* Shanghai, China: Commercial Press.

Stagl, J. (1981). Die Beschreibung des Fremden in der Wissenschaft. In H. P. Duerr (Hg.), *Der Wissenschaftler und das Irrationale. 1.Bd* (pp. 273–295). Frankfurt, Germany: Syndikat Verlag.

Uzarewicz, C., & Uzarewicz, M. (1998). *Kollektive Identität und Tod. Zur Bedeutung ethnischer und nationaler Konstruktionen.* Frankfurt, Germany: Peter Lang Verlag.

Weber, M. (1980). *Wirtschaft und Gesellschaft.* Tübingen, Germany: J.C.B. Mohr Verlag.

Weinrich, H. (1990). Wie fern ist die Fremde? Von der Hermeneutik zur interkulturellen Fremdheitsforschung. In D. Krusche & A. Wierlacher (Hg), *Hermeneutik der Fremde* (pp. 48–50). München, Germany: Indicum Verlag.

7

The Concept of Holism

Hesook Suzie Kim

Nursing has been enchanted with the notions of wholeness, holistic, and holism both in practice and theory throughout its modern development. However, the meanings of these terms in nursing varied from context to context and from one period to the next as these themes were introduced into nursing practice and nursing theory with different motivations and perspectives. These terms are used to depict health conceptualizations, approaches toward health, nursing philosophy, ontological orientations, and theoretical perspectives, creating a great deal of confusion in the nursing discourse. There are at least three specific sources of discourse in nursing that created this scene.

The first wave of discourse occurred in the context of nursing practice. Holistic advocacy in nursing has been traced to Nightingale by Shealy (1985), who found in the pioneer's work a promotion for holistic principles applied to the care of the whole patient. The whole patient approach emphasizes the need to consider the patient in terms of body, mind, and spirit, and in the person's "wholistic" relations to environment. Although this orientation stayed within nursing as a foundational idea, it is not until after the World War II that a more sustaining wave of holistic emphasis appeared in nursing. In the 1950s and 1960s, especially in the United States, the idea of holistic nursing philosophy was advocated by many nursing leaders as the way to differentiate nursing from medicine in the form of comprehensive nursing care. The holistic nursing philosophy encompassing comprehensive nursing care was a position developed to orient nursing to focus on all aspects of the patient (including physical, psychological, social, and spiritual) in providing nursing care. This was seen as a departure from the biomedical focus of medicine that was viewed to be reductionistic and oriented to disease and pathology rather than patients as persons. This notion of holism has been integrated into the central ideology of nursing that is often used as a slogan for nursing practice and nursing conceptualizations.

The second wave can be identified with the general holistic health movement, which arose during the late 1960s and 1970s with the sprouting of counterculture and new-age cultures. Rethinking of the ideas of health, illness, and healthy living led to terms such as holistic health, holistic care, holistic nursing, and holistic medicine, which gave a different meaning to the term holistic. *Holistic* within this holistic health movement meant alternative therapies and healing practices that are not based on the traditional biomedicine and natural sciences (Williams, 1998).

Holistic views in this sense are based on the philosophy that emphasizes the integration of body, mind, and spirit as the ground for healing, a multidimensional approach to health practice, and the rejection of an authoritarian approach to health care (Deliman & Smolowe, 1982; Lowenberg, 1989). Although in a generic sense these terms used in this context align with the philosophy of holism that views humans as unified wholes composed of many dimensions functioning interdependently, because they are so often used in conjunction with alternative therapies such as meditation, homeopathy, spiritual healing, touch therapy, imagery, and art therapy these terms have come to have a very specific meaning when used as an adjective in association with health, nursing, medicine, practice and care.

The term holism on the other hand, appeared in the nursing discourse in relation to nursing theory development that began in earnest in the 1970s. Nearly all of the major nursing theorists of the time such as Rogers, Orem, Roy, Newman, Parse, King, and Neuman, regardless of their theoretical perspectives, espoused the holistic philosophy when they were writing about their theories or implications of their theories for nursing practice. This brought on much confusion in sorting out which theorists have holism as their theories' orientations. This confusion was partly handled by Parse, who differentiated nursing theories into simultaneity and totality paradigms (Parse, 1987), bypassing a judgment on holism. Owen and Holmes (1993) include Rogers, Levine, Parse, Watson, and Newman as those espousing holistic concepts in their theoretical work. There are other claims of holism in nursing theories such as by Hudson (1988), Sarter (1988), and Schultz (1987). However, the versions of holism or the tenets of different holisms these authors hold are so varied and unclear that it is difficult who among them are qualified to be holists. Parse, for example, has adopted several concepts from the Rogerian holism such as unitary being, multidimensionality, and evolutionary process.

However, Parse's theory can be viewed to be more centrally rooted within the existential phenomenological ontology. Newman, who began her theoretical work with the Rogerian framework, is moving toward existential phenomenology and spiritualism, although maintaining some tenets of holism. Watson's theory also can be considered not to be espousing the mainstream holism from the ontological point of view (Owen & Holmes, 1993). Of these theorists, Rogers' work is considered in this chapter to discuss and raise questions about how holism is integrated into a theory as an ontological and epistemological orientation.

HOLISM: DEFINITIONS, PHILOSOPHICAL ORIENTATIONS, AND VARIETIES

The term, holism, is a combination of *hol-* or *holo-* meaning complete, entire, without division, or whole and *ism*, suggesting an ideology of wholes. Holism as a term has been attributed to Jan C. Smuts, a South African politician and statesman, as its first formal user in 1926 (Smuts, 1926). It refers in its simplistic sense to a philosophy that the nature or the universe needs to be viewed in terms of wholes that are irreducible to parts and are more than the sum of their parts. However, philosophically, the term conveys much more complex ideas, including not only the irreducibility of wholes to parts and the wholistic unity but also evolution and emergence as the basic features of wholes. Inherent in some holisms are specific ideas regarding the wholes' relations with their environment and hierarchical relations among the wholes. Holism has been applied in the conceptualizations and studies of not only living organisms including humans, but also physical systems, social institutions including societies and cultures, nature, and even the universe as a unity. Such diverse philosophies underpinning holism, some interrelated and others providing distinct perspectives, make a discussion of holism in the nursing context problematic.

Holism or holistic idea is viewed by many scholars to have a long history, some tracing its roots back to the classical Greek period, with continuing transformations through the eighteenth and nineteenth centuries and most intensely in the current century. Holism as it developed at the close of the nineteenth century and in the wake of the twentieth century was a response to the reductionism, mechanism, and atomism that were becoming the dominant scientific philosophies not only for the so-called natural, hard sciences such as physics, chemistry, and biology, but also in psychology, sociology, anthropology, and political sciences. Hence, scientific holism was a development to challenge the adequacies of various scientific approaches such as mechanism, reductionism, atomism, and dualism. This movement against reductionism, mechanism, and atomism responded with various alternative forms of holism to consider units (be they biological organisms, institutions, societies, or political entities) as wholes and study them as *whole qua whole*. In this sense, scientific holism has risen with a unified agenda but developed into multiple types and forms.

There are various ways of differentiating types of holisms. Phillips (1976) traces the development of holism in terms of three types: *holism 1*, *holism 2*, and *holism 3* in relation to their oppositions to mechanistic (analytic) method, reductionism, and atomism. His arguments are directed to critiquing the epistemological bases of holisms, rather than the holism's ontology. Phillips identifies *holism 1* as organicism representing a set of five interrelated ideas regarding organic wholes, which are, for Phillips, the starting points for discussing three types of holism:

1. The analytic approach as typified by the physicochemical sciences proves inadequate when applied to certain cases—for example, to a biological organism, to society, or even to reality as a whole.
2. The whole is more than the sum of its parts.
3. The whole determines the nature of its parts.
4. The parts cannot be understood if considered in isolation from the whole.
5. The parts are dynamically related or interdependent (Phillips, 1976, p. 6).

Phillips suggests that all of these characteristics of *holism 1* are logically based on the Hegelian theory of internal relations set against the mechanistic (analytic) method of science (1976, pp. 6–20). Hence, Phillips' *holism 1* was a development that connects the ontology of holism with the theory of internal relations as its basis of epistemology. Phillips acknowledges that *holism 1* in its original form as biological organicism changed into a much more complex notion after about 1930 (1976, p. 29). According to Phillips, *holism 2* emerged with a specifically antireductionistic agenda with the major thesis that "the properties of organic wholes or systems, *after* they have been found, cannot be explained in terms of the properties of the parts" (1976, p. 34). *Holism 2* is seen to be specifically opposed to the methodological individualism of Popper and other social scientists. On the other hand, *holism 3* espouses that "it is necessary to have terms referring to whole and their properties" (p. 37). This thesis finds support in the holism of general system theory of Bertalanffy (1969) and Koestler (1967). Phillips, through his analysis of various forms of holistic theories within the tradition of holism, which includes biological organicism, general system theory, functionalism, structuralism, and gestalt psychology, concludes that it is generally correct about the holists' positions regarding (a) the emphasis on the dynamic relation between the parts of an organic whole, (b) the idea that it is difficult to predict emerging properties through the study of parts, and (c) the notion that new concepts are necessary to study organic wholes scientifically. However, the holists are wrong to think "that there is anything here that is antithetical to the traditional analytic (or atomistic, or reductionistic) method" (Phillips, 1976, p. 123). He also concludes that holism is "an eminently unworkable doctrine" (p. 123). Hence, he disputes the validity of the holism's epistemological foundation and suggests that logically there is nothing that should deter holists to use the analytic or mechanistic method in the study of wholes.

In a different perspective, Harrington (1996) identifies several different origins of holism as a philosophy that sprang against the growing "disenchantment" with the mechanistic scientific ethos of the early twentieth century. She saw this holistic science not as a movement based on a single perspective but as "a family of approaches" of which the central tenet was "the need to do justice to organismic purposiveness or teleological functioning" (Harrington, 1996, p. xvii). Different holistic approaches were developed with varying commitments to the ideas that (a) organisms must be viewed not as mere sums of their elementary parts and processes but as wholes having distinct characteristics as wholes; (b) the ontological categories of humans as body and mind as in dualism must be rejected, and humans must be considered as wholes and studied as wholes; (c) organismic or systemic processes for any given system must be viewed in the context of a larger system or the universe; and (d) the mechanistic science (the machine science) must be rejected with the new science of wholeness for the humanity to regain its true dignity (Harrington, 1996, pp. xvii–xix). Harrington sees this new holistic science of life and mind having influences not only as a "more authentic vision of life and mind" with which knowledge in biology, psychology, and sociology was developing in new directions but also as a "blueprint for visualizing" a more authentic future in the political arena (Harrington, 1995, 1996). Hence, unlike Phillips, Harrington offers a view of holism from its penetration into the collective, cultural life in a historical context. Under the guise of holistic thinking the twentieth century is entrenched with diverse and somewhat paradoxical development of such political and cultural ideologies as totalitarianism, political unitarism, and cultural determinism as well as a movement toward humanistic ideologies.

Several other ways of differentiating holism can point to the variety of terms used to describe differences in holisms. From the perspective of environmental ethics, Marietta (1995) proposes three forms of holism: (a) biocentric holism in which all living things are considered to be wholes living with the natural environment, (b) ecocentric holism or environmental holism that views the natural system as a whole, and (c) holistic anthropocentrism that recognizes humans as a part of nature but also as a distinct holistic entity. On a different note, James (1984) differentiates holism of content from holism of form from a sociological perspective. Holism of content is advocated by social theorists who view the characteristics of social wholes to be qualitatively distinct from the characteristics of their parts, insisting that social theories must incorporate the ontology of social wholes in their explanations. On the other hand, holism of form is epistemologically oriented, and is a view that each term in a theory "owes its meaning to its relations with the others" (James, 1984, p. 3). This means that all terms of theories are defined in relation to each other and within the given theories. Holism thus is viewed separately, although it can be related in important ways, from either the ontological or the epistemological stance.

Again from a sociological perspective, Chattopadhyaya (1967) offers different versions of holism as biological organicism, idealistic organicism, psychological organicism, functionalism, and structural-functionalism, all of which are seen to adhere to the notion that human actions must be explained in the appropriate social context as a whole. Täljedal (1997) offers yet another set of terminology to differentiate versions of holism in medicine and medical sociology: strong and weak holisms. According to him, strong holism is based on the "layer ontology" of viewing human beings constituted by a set of distinct but integrative levels of organization, whereas weak holism espouses conceptualizations of health in the context of individuals as wholes. These are similar to Kolcaba's (1997) differentiation of holism into systemic holism, organismic holism, and whole-person holism, all of which are based on the ways patients are conceptualized. Viewing none of these versions satisfactory for nursing, he suggests person-based holism as the solution to consolidate systemic and organismic holisms with the whole-person holism as an ecumenical way of handling knowledge development in nursing (Kolcaba, 1997).

In all of this diversity in holism and holistic philosophy, there are four influential and sustaining themes coming from several eminent scientists and philosophers. First, this is based on the tenets of organicism that evolved into viewing an organism as a whole that has functional relationships with its environment. Organicism also introduced the idea of teleology as the basis of the whole organism's survival, growth, and change.

The second theme comes from General System Theory (GST) of Bertalanffy and Koestler's hierarchical conceptualization of systems. The major tenets of GST as a general science of wholeness include the concept of system as organized wholes of which elements are interdependent and in mutual interaction and the principles of emergence, entropy and negentropy, equifinality, and so forth applicable to systems regardless of the nature of parts and their relationships among the parts (Bertalanffy, 1969). Added to these notions of GST is the concept of open hierarchical systems of Koestler, of which he states that "[w]hat we find are intermediary structures on a series of levels in an ascending order of complexity: subwholes which display, according to the way you look at them, some of the characteristics commonly attributed to wholes and some of the characteristics commonly attributed to parts" (Koestler, 1967, p. 48). Inherent in this conceptualization of hierarchy is the idea that there is no entity that is fundamentally a part or a whole except when the entities are considered in relation to one another. Entities therefore are "subordinated as *parts* to the higher centers in the hierarchy, but at the same time function as quasi-autonomous *wholes*. They are Janus-faced. The face turned upward, toward the higher levels, is that of a dependent part; the face turned downward, towards its own constituents, is that of a whole of remarkable self-sufficiency" (Koestler, 1978, p. 27). These systems-based ideas for holism thus do not require holists to use organismic metaphors in addressing wholes as units of analysis.

The third theme undergirding various holisms comes from the idea of evolution, drawing from Darwin's inspiring work that changed the way scientists looked at life, development, and change. In holism, Teilhard de Chardin's evolutionary ideas are cited often. Teilhard de Chardin (1959) espoused that humans as well as other entities are constantly evolving toward progressively higher, more complex and sophisticated, and more perfectly unified entities. Although the evolutionism of Teilhard de Chardin was oriented to the final point of evolution in the unity of humanity and the nature with God, the idea of evolution as a holistic one undercuts many versions of holism.

The fourth theme is related to the thinking that unites all things, all of reality as a whole. David Bohm's version of holism, which may be termed as universal holism, is based on the idea that the phenomena of the universe need to be expressed in terms of wholeness and movement (Bohm, 1980). In his conceptualization of the universal holism, Bohm states that " . . . each particle is only an abstraction of a relatively invariant form of movement in the whole field of the universe" and that "elementary particles are on-going movements that are mutually dependent because ultimately they merge and interpenetrate" (1980, p. 29). His version of holism thus relates the wholeness to the entire reality uniting it with what he calls holomovement.

It is evident then that holisms (not as a singular philosophy but as multiple, different philosophies), both from the ontological and epistemological contexts, are based on many ideas. None of the holisms espoused either by philosophers or scientists endorses all tenets that are considered to be related to holism. The following are the major ideas that can undergird various holisms:

- An entity is considered a whole when it is composed of parts that are interdependent and in mutual interaction.
- Wholeness is inherent in reality and is the essential character of entities.
- The whole is more than the sum of its parts and is distinct in its characteristics from its parts.
- The whole determines the nature of its parts, and the parts have ontological significance in the context of the whole.
- The whole is an emergent entity and follows evolutionary processes toward increasing complexity and diversity.
- An entity as a whole is in constant interaction with its environment.
- An entity as a whole is embedded in a larger whole in that all entities as wholes are organized in a hierarchical level of interaction and interdependence.
- There are distinct principles that govern the behaviors and characteristics of wholes, which are only applicable to wholes.

While it is possible to categorize holism in many different versions, as seen in the preceding section, for the purpose of exposition in nursing, four types that endorse various combinations of the above holistic ideas are identified as entitative holism, anthropocentric holism, hierarchical systemic holism, and universal cosmic holism. The differences among these holisms are depicted in Figure 7.1.

Entitative holism is a position that considers living and nonliving entities of reality to be wholes. Each class of entity as a whole possesses its unique characteristics that are different from its constituent parts, and are governed by specific sets of holistic processes that define its behaviors as a whole unit. Within this holism, different holistic entities are viewed

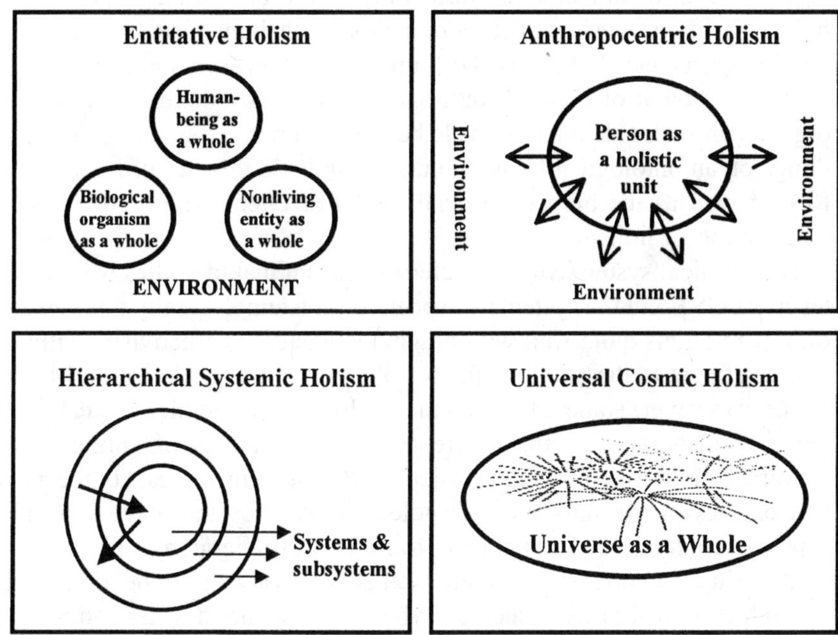

FIGURE 7.1. Representation of different types of holism.

to be governed by explanatory principles of change and behaviors that may be unique. This form of holism aligns with the scientific holism that opposes reductionism and atomism, but not necessarily mechanism.

Anthropocentric holism is holism that focuses on humans as holistic units with characteristics and processes distinct from other animate and inanimate entities of the world. This version of holism highlights the interpenetrating, interdependent nature of body, mind, and spirit (soul) as a whole. It also views humans to have a distinct holistic character that is different from other entities of the world and unique in itself. Humans as wholes are in interaction with the environment, however, the environment is not necessarily considered to be a whole itself or composed of other types of wholes. In this holism, human beings exist, experience, and behave as wholes through the processes that unite and integrate all aspects of human beings. Illness thus is explained not in terms of an elevated blood sugar level or an enlarged cardiac valve, but in terms of the individual's state or experience that results from the integration of such phenomenon through holistic processes. Humans' relationships with their environment are viewed either as complementary and interdependent or as controlling and selective through human processes. This version of holism is often considered in conjunction with humanism, because the ontological center in both is the humans. Gestalt psychology is in line with this version of holism. Anthropocentric holism therefore is akin to organicism with a distinction made between humans from all other living things on an ontological basis. In nursing, holistic theories of Levine and Roy as well as the biopsychosocial model of clients align closely with this version of holism.

Hierarchical systemic holism refers to holism that identifies with many tenets of GST and the systems perspective. Epistemologically this version of holism aligns quite well with pragmatism and constructivism, without a commitment to the ontology that wholeness is inherent in entities themselves. However, some adherents may subscribe to the hierarchical, systemic characteristic as the inherent and true features of entities in a universal system of systems. Basically, this holism represents the idea that entities of the universe as wholes are systems that have sub- and supersystem relations among them, forming into a hierarchy. Hierarchical relationships among systems are sometimes viewed to be organized through a control process such as cybernetics, while they are sometimes considered to be in interdependent relationships. However, the notion of hierarchy suggests an attribution of whole to the unit having the point of attention at the analytic moment while that same unit becomes a part of a higher level unit (or system) when the point of attention is shifted to that higher level. Hence, an entity as a system is a whole and not a whole depending on how that entity is viewed or analyzed. Because of this, within this version of holism parts are referred to as subsystems holding all characteristics of a system at their levels of analysis. Talcott Parsons' theory of social system (1951) aligns with this version in sociology. In nursing the conceptual models of King, Roy, and Neuman partly align with this version.

Universal cosmic holism is the holism adhering to the notion that the universe in its totality is a whole, organized through processes that unite and integrate all elements contained within the universe to emerge and change as a whole. The universe is seen to possess a unitary pattern that permeates and interpenetrating in all elements. The processes of the universe are often expressed in terms of multidimensionality, evolution and emergence toward increasing complexity and diversity, and unity. In this model, humans are integral parts of the universe, inseparable and connected within the universal character. Humans as well as all separate entities, living and nonliving, must be understood in terms of the universe, in the image of the total cosmos. In that sense, humans lose their unique features. Morowitz states in the same context that "[e]ach living thing is a dissipative structure, that is, it does not endure in and of itself but only as a results of the continual flow in the system" (1972, p. 156). This points to the possibility of holism leading to a different kind of reduction. Ecological holism, which is in line with this version, has been viewed to be "totalitarian" (Kheel, 1985) and to project a "fascist understanding of the environment" (Regan, 1981). The picture of this universal cosmic holism is well depicted in Francis Thompson's poem that says "thou canst not stir a flower/Without troubling of a star." The major tenets of this holism are interconnectedness of all elements of the universe and the interpenetration of the universal patterns in all elements unifying them into one unitary movement such as the concept of holomovement espoused by Bohm. Martha Rogers' science of unitary human beings adopts some of the tenets of this version of holism.

What I have discussed so far points to the diversity in the philosophy of holism, and the possible difficulty with which one can judge a theory or conceptual model to be truly holistic. However, there are also other fundamental issues associated with the philosophy of holism as the foundation for science and scientific work from an epistemological stance. There are at least three issues that pose difficulties in developing science from the holistic philosophy: (a) difficulties in developing explanations in terms of *whole qua whole*, (b) the issue of holistic reduction, and (c) problems of method in relation to conceptualization and measurement. First, while there are several theoretical principles in holism associated with the fundamental tenets identified earlier, theoreticians are finding it difficult to develop explanations of behaviors or states of wholes through the explication of holistic processes. Theoretically, holistic processes are often identifiable only descriptively, without pointing to explanations of holistic behaviors or states. Second, on the other hand, holistic theories may lead to reduction of a kind that is different from the physical reductionism. Holistic reduction prevents views and understandings of human experiences from particular, distinct orientations, especially when humans are considered parts in ecocentric or universal holism (Gadow, 1992). Third, because one of the major tenets of holism is in conceptualizing wholes as uniquely wholes and not in terms of parts, it is necessary to conceptualize holistic phenomena with new language (as specified in Phillips' holism 3). This means that there is a need for a unified science, for example for all of the sciences that deal with humans or living organisms, or even for all sciences, united by a new set of scientific language and general theoretical principles. Holism with the stance against analytic reductionism and decomposition must come up with concepts that specify phenomena of wholes. For example, human phenomena in holism then would need to be conceptualized not from the biological, psychological, social, or nursing perspectives because such perspectives would only be addressing partial views, but from a unified, holistic perspective. Holism points to a perspectiveless science, thus a new way of defining different scientific disciplines must then be developed within holism. This is a challenge that cannot be taken lightly.

ROGERS' SCIENCE OF UNITARY HUMAN BEINGS

Rogers' science of unitary human beings as a theoretical framework was first proposed in 1970, has gone through several stages of conceptual and theoretical revisions. The theory, as it was proposed in 1970 and labeled as "a science of unitary man" in 1980, had a strong alliance with the holism of general system theory, especially that of Bertalanffy, field theory, and the general evolutionary tenets (Rogers, 1970, and 1980). From these, she adopted the notions of humans as open systems and complex energy fields. The concept of energy field refers to the entitative feature of humans and environment, meaning that humans and environment are "energy fields" rather than humans and environment have energy. The pattern of energy field was depicted as "a mosaic of waves" in her earlier work, but later referred to as a single wave. She also conceptualized humans as "a unified whole possessing his own integrity and manifesting characteristics that are more than and different from the sum of his parts" (Rogers, 1970, p. 47). By 1983, Rogers emphasized the irreducibility of the human energy field, a concept that she viewed to represent her paradigm to be "unitary" rather than "holistic." In 1970, she embraced the notion that "man and environment are continuously exchanging matter and energy with one another" (Rogers, 1970, p. 54), but later dropped this "exchange assumption" completely. The idea of mutual process and integration of the human and environment energy fields replaced it.

Rogers conceptualized human beings as continuously changing their life patterns (patterning) toward increasing complexity and negentropy. Life patterning is viewed in terms of the wholeness of the unitary human being expressed as the human energy field. The patterns of life processes are seen as manifested through the unitary human being's mutual, simultaneous integrating process with the environment through the principles of homeodynamics specified as helicy, resonancy, synchrony, and reciprocity. The principles of synchrony and reciprocity were combined into the principle of complementarity, which later became the principle of integrality.

Rogers also began her conceptualization of negentropic journey in a linear space-time notion, but later anchored it in multidimensional context. In doing so, she moved toward the universal, cosmic holism: " . . . the integrality of people and their environments coordinates with a pandimensional universe of open systems, point to a new paradigm . . . " (Rogers, 1992, p. 28). By 1992, Rogers had moved to view her framework to be rooted in a pandimensional view of people and their world, moving beyond the usual notions of multidimensionality of universal existence. As specified by Rogers' writings of 1992, Rogers' science of unitary human beings are based on the following assumptions and conceptualizations:

- A pandimensional worldview is a way of perceiving reality within a universe of open systems. Hence, all reality is pandimensional. Pandimensionality refers to "an infinite domain without limit" that is nonlinear and without spatial or temporal attributes. Pandimensionality "expresses the idea of a unitary whole" (Rogers, 1992, p. 31).
- Within this view, the fundamental units of both the living and the nonliving are energy fields that are infinite, pandimensional, and in continuous motion. An energy field is perceived as a single wave. The human energy field and the environmental energy field are identified as distinct fields. The human energy field can be conceptualized for a single human being or groups by which either an individual or a group is considered irreducible and indivisible, once they are conceptualized as a singular unit. Each human energy field (either as a singular individual or a group) is integral with its own environmental field that is unique to it.
- Both human beings and their respective environments are unitary and irreducible wholes.
- The distinguishing characteristic of an energy field perceived as a single wave is patterning that eventuates from the mutual process of the human-environmental fields based on the principles of homeodynamics (of resonancy, helicy, and integrality). Field patterning is characterized by change that is continuous, relative, innovative, creative, increasingly diverse, and unpredictable.
- Field patterning is emergent and unpredictable. Causality is rejected.
- "The evolution of life and nonlife is a dynamic, irreducible, nonlinear process characterized by increasing complexification of energy field patterning" (Rogers, 1992, p. 31). Hence, all entities in the universe follow this evolutionary process.
- Nursing based on a science of unitary human beings is "inseparable from the new world view and the process of change," (Rogers, 1992,

p. 33) and the phenomena of concern for nursing from this view are people and their world in a pandimensional universe.

What are the essences of Rogers' epistemology and her holism then? Rogers' epistemological position for her science of unitary human beings is constructivism in which the conceptualization and language of the science are viewed to be constructions to make the subject matter unique to nursing. She stressed that the definitions, meanings, and principles of her science are only valid within the context of the science of unitary human beings. Rogers was also a perspectivist because she acknowledged the legitimacy of viewing humans and environments in other ways, especially from other disciplinary perspectives, than the one she espoused, that is, the study of unitary, irreducible, indivisible human and environmental fields as the unique focus of nursing. Hence, to Rogers, humans possess many distinct characteristics that may be conceptualized differently according to specific disciplines' foci of attention. To her, nursing's phenomena of concern need to be people and their environments conceptualized in a pandimensional worldview as unitary, irreducible, indivisible human and environmental fields. Why this must be so, she did not say. She insisted that this is a unique way for nursing to conceptualize its subject matter.

Rogers' position on holism is a paradoxical one: she suggested that the term holistic not be used to indicate her notion of unitary human beings in her later writings, and yet she believed that her worldview is holistic. One of the important assertions of Rogers is the negation of parts in wholes. The notion of parts is irrelevant within the concept of unitary wholes that are irreducible and indivisible. Hence, there are no parts identifiable in wholes to Rogers. This is a departure from the general positions of holism that acknowledges the existence or possibility of parts within wholes, but aligns with David Bohm's idea that fragmentation results from the way of seeing the universe and is not the essential character of the holistic universe. In addition, she embraced various aspects of the entitative holism, anthropocentric holism, and universal cosmic holism without reconciling the diverse orientations these three versions of holism support.

Rogers viewed unitary human beings and unitary environments as distinct fields within a universe of open systems, suggesting that a universe is constituted by fields considered to be wholes. Fields as wholes are viewed to be irreducible and indivisible. She also suggested that all entities (living and nonliving) change in an evolutionary sense in a dynamic, irreducible, and nonlinear process. These views align with the tenets of the entitative holism. However, Rogers' conceptualization of field as the fundamental holistic unit is arbitrary and fluid. This means that her notion of field may refer to entities that have specific boundaries such as human beings as well as those that are defined as fields when analytic needs arise. Environments as fields are relative to the focused human fields. This means that an environmental field relative to one specific human field embraces other human fields into an irreducible, indivisible whole that is the respective environmental field. If each and every human field is unitary, is it possible for any human field to be completely embedded into an environmental field of another human being to lose its identity as a unitary being? If this is so, then how is it possible for one human field to retain its unitary wholeness, while it is also possible for it to be embraced into an irreducible, indivisible environmental field? In discussing the theory of accelerating evolution derived from Rogers' science of unitary human beings, Rogers seemed to suggest the environmental field as a nonhuman field. If this is the case, then Rogers' environmental field must be conceptualized to be devoid of humans. Both conceptualizations of environmental field, one that embraces all other humans and the other excluding humans, present logical problems in relation to field patterning and mutual processing. Furthermore, Rogers suggested that unitary human beings as wholes that are conceptualized as irreducible and indivisible at one point may be subsumed within other wholes that are irreducible and indivisible at another point. For example, the conceptualization of family energy field or crowd as an energy field. This relative conceptualization of field and the specific identification of human energy field and environmental energy field point to various logical problems.

On the other hand, Rogers' focus is in human beings, of which energy fields are viewed to be unique and in a continuous mutual process with their unique environmental fields. This notion is close to the anthropocentric holism in which the central focus is the humans and their relationships with environment. Rogers also views the human and environmental change and evolution to be interpenetrating, coordinated, and together in a single wave patterning. This view reflecting David Bohm's holism leans toward the universal cosmic holism. This orientation shifts the focus of study from humans to the universe, thus making it difficult to conceptualize the appropriate phenomena of concern for nursing.

Therefore, Rogers' holism is eclectic and contains several points raised above that need to be reconciled. It is an abstract system that needs to be specified further in terms of language and conceptualization as well as through research. In addition, although Rogers indicates that "people's capacity to participate knowingly in the process of change" (1990) is inherent in this science, this idea is not apparent in the conceptualization of field patterning expressed through the principles of homeodynamics. This vision of holism then highlights the integrality of humans and their environment rather than human's proactive (both positive and negative) potential to influence the process of change.

CONCLUSIONS

The concept of holism as examined in this chapter is associated with complex and multiple sets of ideas used as ontological and epistemological bases for science. The term holism is used both casually and seriously in the literature, especially in the nursing literature. Nearly all of the nursing theorists used the term holism or holistic in describing their theories, often without specifying which assumptions of holism are incorporated into their theories. Besides Rogers, whose work was discussed in this chapter, Roy, Newman, Neuman, Parse, Orem, Levine, King, and Watson support one or two of the holistic tenets in their theories and theoretical models. Holism as nursing philosophy and as the basis for theory development in nursing has been in place for a long time. It is difficult to say what future holism has for nursing unless we are able to address why holism is necessary, desirable, essential, or important for nursing conceptualizations and nursing practice. If it is answered from an ontological perspective, holism must be addressed from the way we conceptualize nursing clients as human beings. If it is answered from an epistemological perspective, holism points to new ways of developing knowledge. In nursing, we must also address the question that how significantly holistic nursing theories accommodate essential and important issues of nursing practice. Phillip's despair that "holism is an eminently unworkable doctrine" (1976, p. 123) must be overcome by various logical, empirical, and conceptual means if nursing were to continue with its insistence to hold onto holism as its major orientation.

REFERENCES

Bertalanffy, L. (1969). *General system theory: Foundations, development, applications.* New York: Braziller.

Bohm, D. (1980). *Wholeness and the implicate order.* London: Routledge & Kegan Paul.

Chattopadhyaya, D. (1967). *Individuals and societies: A methodological inquiry.* New York: Allied.

Deliman, T., & Smolowe, J. S. (Eds.). (1982). *Holistic medicine.* Reston, VA: Reston.

Gadow, S. (1992). Existential ecology: The human/natural world. *Social Science and Medicine, 35,* 596–602.

Harrington, A. (1995). Metaphoric connections: Holistic science in the shadow of the Third Reich. *Social Research, 62,* 357–386.

Harrington, A. (1996). *Reenchanted science: Holism in German culture from Wilhelm II to Hitler.* Princeton, NJ: Princeton University Press.

Hudson, R. (1988). Whole or parts: A theoretical perspective on person. *Australian Journal of Advanced Nursing, 6,* 12–20.

James, S. (1984). *The content of social explanation.* Cambridge, UK: Cambridge University Press.

Kheel, M. (1985). The liberation of nature: A circular affair. *Environmental Ethics, 7,* 135–149.

Koestler, A. (1967). *The ghost in the machine.* New York: Macmillan.

Koestler, A. (1978). *Janus: A summing up.* New York: Random House.

Kolcaba, R. (1997). The primary holisms in nursing. *Journal of Advanced Nursing, 25,* 290–296.

Lowenberg, J. S. (1989). *Caring and responsibility: The crossroads between holistic practice and traditional medicine.* Philadelphia: University of Pennsylvania Press.

Marietta, D. Jr. (1995). *For people and the planet: Holism and humanism in environmental ethics.* Philadelphia: Temple University Press.

Morowitz, H. J. (1972). Biology as a cosmological science. *Main Currents in Modern Thought, 28,* 156.

Owen, M. J., & Holmes, C. A. (1993). "Holism" in the discourse of nursing. *Journal of Advanced Nursing, 18,* 1688–1695.

Parse, R. R. (1987). *Nursing science: Major paradigms, theories, and critiques.* Philadelphia: Saunders.

Parsons, T. (1951). *The social system.* New York: The Free Press.

Phillips, D. C. (1976). *Holistic thought in social science.* Stanford, CA: Stanford University Press.

Regan, T. (1981). The nature and possibility of an environmental ethic. *Environmental Ethics, 3,* 19–34.

Rogers, M. E. (1970). *An introduction to the theoretical basis of nursing.* Philadelphia: Davis.

Rogers, M. E. (1980). Nursing: A science of unitary man. In J. P. Riehl & C. Roy (Eds.), *Conceptual models for nursing practice* (2nd ed., pp. 329–337). New York: Appleton-Century-Crofts.

Rogers, M. E. (1990). Nursing: science of unitary, irreducible, human beings: Update 1990. In E. A. M. Barrett (Ed.), *Visions of Rogers' science-based nursing* (pp. 5–11). New York: National League for Nursing.

Rogers, M. E. (1992). Nursing science and the space age. *Nursing Science Quarterly, 5,* 27–34.

Sarter, B. (1988). Philosophical sources of nursing theory. *Nursing Science Quarterly, 1,* 52–59.

Schultz, P. R. (1987). Toward holistic inquiry in nursing. A proposal for synthesis of patterns and methods. *Scholarly Inquiry for Nursing Practice: An International Journal, 1,* 135–146.

Shealy, M. C. (1985). Florence Nightingale 1820–1910: An evolutionary mind in the context of holism. *Journal of Holistic Nursing Practice, 3,* 4–6.

Smuts, J. C. (1926). *Holism and evolution.* London: Oxford University Press.

Täljedal, I. (1997). Weak and strong holism. *Scandinavian Journal of Social Medicine, 25,* 67–69.

Teilhard de Chardin, P. (1959) *The phenomenon of man, with an introduction by Sir Julian Huxley.* New York: Harper & Row.

Williams, A. (1998). Therapeutic landscapes in holistic medicine. *Social Science and Medicine, 46,* 1193–1203.

8

Applying Social Science Concepts to Nursing: Systems Theory and Beyond*

Jens Friebe

This chapter takes a look at the two scientific fields of nursing science and social science; using examples, it then examines the basic features of systems approaches to nursing theory before finally presenting topics for further reflections on nursing.

SYSTEMS PERSPECTIVES IN NURSING SCIENCE AND SOCIAL SCIENCES

The contribution of the social sciences to nursing science is often focused on in current discussions, whereby three lines of argumentation emerge:

- Discarding the medical paradigm of nursing raises the question of the extent to which the social sciences have a share in the construction of a separate and independent nursing paradigm;
- sociological systems theory is an integral part of a number of nursing theories; sociological phase theories, on the other hand, have been given little consideration; and
- social science research methods are of great value to nursing science.

The discussion of the significance of key paradigms (which belongs more appropriately to the theory of science but which in nursing science discourse was sparked in particular by the contributions of Fawcett [1995]) is not to be given any special consideration here because links and relation-

*Translated from German by Gerald Nixon.

ships between individual scientific disciplines and nursing are better analysed at the level of short- and medium-range theories. Although general systems theory and cybernetics have certainly found their way into numerous approaches to nursing theory, their influences and adaptations first become manifest when one looks at what has actually been borrowed from systems-based sociology or social psychology. What is conspicuous here is that frequently under the heading nursing and social science quite different things are compared because the social science perspective is sometimes considered to embrace everything not belonging to the natural sciences or used as an undefined collective term for sociology, psychology, pedagogic, economics, and other scientific fields. In this chapter the argumentation is thus limited to theories concerning human action in groups and institutions.

The concept of systems originated in comparative studies of mathematics, biology, physics, and the social sciences: "By system we mean in a very general sense a set of elements which stand in relation to one another, are regarded as a unit and can be marked off from their environment" (Siegrist, 1988, p. 85). Systems and subsystems can be differentiated according to duration, density, and magnitude. They react to influences from their environment by compensating for differences between what ought to be and what actually is with the aim of achieving stability and equilibrium. Cybernetics, as the study of the art of steering transcending the scientific disciplines, has provided numerous examples of systems processes: in physics, feedback control systems, which, for instance, regulate the central heating in a house; in biology, body processes such as yawning owing to a lack of oxygen; in economics, competition leading to certain spatial structures (the Chicago school) or, in the social sciences, the balance between personal and group identities.

In the wake of the "gradual process of scientification" (Schaeffer, Moers, & Rosenbrock, 1994) the nursing theories from the United States that have become familiar in Germany provide a link between nursing science and sociological systems theory. This is not surprising, bearing in mind that Parsons once suggested that the term sociology be replaced by the term systems theory (Korte, 1993, p. 178). Social systems were described by Parsons as "states and processes of social interaction between acting units" (Parsons, 1971, p. 7) that reveal an organizational structure in their subsystems and special relationships with their environment. Subsystems, organisms, personal, social, and cultural systems and their functions of adaptation, goal attainment, integration and structure maintenance—all of which are defined by Parsons—are also the basic categories employed in nursing theories (King, 1981).

The European social sciences, on the other hand, have brought forth outstanding theories of phases and processes dealing with the change of society rather than with the preservation of its structures. Examples of this are provided by, among others, Auguste Comte, Karl Marx, Max Weber, and Norbert Elias. It is not intended here to take up the discussion of so-called wide-ranging sociological theories; what is intended, however, is to place the focus of the investigation on social change. Today, sociology is at great pains to do away with the dualisms that have long dominated thinking. The issue is not whether systems or processes are observed as the synchronic or diachronic perspectives but rather how the transformation of systems in and through time occurs. It is no longer a question of tradition or modernity but rather of the simultaneity of the unsimultaneous. It is not a matter of social stratum/class or individual/relations, but it is as Bourdieu expressed it in his question: "Which system of classification and evaluation do the actors use, and in what relationship do they stand to the social classes?" (Bourdieu, 1993, p. 51). Thus, the task of sociology is to put the actions of individuals and groups in relation to the structures—to link the micro and the macro perspectives (the worm's and the bird's eye views) in a meaningful way.

As Johnson (1980) has posited, although nursing theories may be borrowed, they are nevertheless unique. The borrowing took place at a certain time in scientific development and the loans are now arriving in Germany only after considerable delay. As a result, further advances in the knowledge gathered in the social sciences, for example in systems theory in sociology or behavioral theory in psychology, have not been taken into account in nursing theory approaches. Researchers such as Johnson, King, Roy, and Neuman borrowed concepts for their theories in an early period of the development of systems theory, thus scarcely questioning the goal of adapting individual behavior to societal conditions. Johnson, for example, considers the task of nursing to be maintaining the equilibrium in the behavior system; for Roy it is helping the individual to adjust to wellness and illness; whereas King sees it as ensuring that people function in their social roles (Fawcett, 1995). This way of thinking may certainly be meaningfully applied in specific nursing situations or in fulfilling management tasks. Yet the functional perspective of this thinking becomes clear only when one takes into considerations that it is frequently based on a complementary distribution of roles between nursing staff and patients, that there is no discussion of their interactional relationship, and that the unobservable impulses of behavior as well as changes in personal circumstances are completely ignored.

What is the role of nursing and what is its status in a complex society in which the service sector is gaining increasing importance? These are questions that are not easily answered because different models of society must be taken into account in the analysis. If one assumes that modern societies are service societies, characterized among other things by differentiation, individualism, and mobility, attention to the individual client will be given a prominent place in nursing. If, on the other hand, it is assumed that now as before societies are dominated by dimensions of inequality (two-thirds/one-third societies), then the tasks of the nursing staff will have to be defined as change agents. In the final analysis, the synthesis of nursing science and social science will always have to be examined in accordance with the criteria of the prevailing ideology. A theory of goal attainment will have to answer questions as to whose goals and whose interests have been used to set the norms to go beyond merely satisfying the requirements of external control or, as Kim has expressed it: "Is the primary goal of nursing science in understanding or in control?" (Kim, 1989, p. 108).

SYSTEMS APPROACHES IN NURSING THEORY

Johnson (1980) describes nursing as a regulative force that becomes necessary when defects occur in the structure of a system or subsystem. The aim of nursing is to contribute through "the fostering of efficient and effective behavioral functioning in the patient to prevent illness, and during and following illness" (Johnson, 1980, p. 207). The behavioral system is stimulated to respond by means of stressors, leading to action involving the seven named subsystems and patterns of behavior. If these are not sufficient to deal with the stress functionally, this may be an indication that regulation is required through nursing with the aim of protecting, stimulating, and furthering the individual. This model thus represents an adaptation of Parson's systems model and Selye's behaviorist stress model (1956). However, it was not long before Lazarus pointed out that Selye's view of stress was one-sided because perception of stress and response depended just as much on cognition and emotion as they did linearly on stimuli (Zimbardo, 1995, p. 580). Cognition and emotion were aspects to which Selye, a zoologist, had given less consideration. Consequently, although Johnson's reflections have broadened the scope of observation in nursing in important areas, the analysis of psychical and interactional relationships remains an unresolved question.

King attempted to overcome these inadequacies by formulating a superordinate frame of reference for nursing as well as a theory of goal attainment. As a conceptual model, King's general systems model is meant to provide room for different theories, all of which are holistically related to the personal, interpersonal, and social systems. She writes: "The artificial boundaries of nursing are individuals and groups interacting with the environment" (King, 1981, p. 1). She thus judges that her model solves the problems of inadequate connection with social interaction and insufficient differentiation of within and without, the individual and the environment, inherent in other systems models. In King's framework, while the question of individual and environment is solved by making either the person or the group/society a system in hierarchical relations with the environment, interaction is given a separate approach in the form of the theory of goal attainment. In the encounter between nurse and patient key categories of social psychology such as perception, judgment, and response are used to analyze an interactional relationship. The term transaction, signifying intentional, goal-oriented behavior, is introduced as a category, which is meant to give an exact description of the work involved in nursing (King, 1981, 1995). Furthermore, the theory of goal attainment is linked to the model of the nursing process and nursing diagnoses. Here, one might ask what the profile of a theory is that apparently integrates all approaches, be they from the social sciences or from nursing science. The theory fails to meet its own demand of focusing on social interaction because dynamic developments and differing symmetries in human relationships are given no consideration so that in the end one arrives at the conclusion that nursing is made up of interactions, the immediately observable part of which can be represented using the means at the disposal of cognitive psychology.

The attempt to establish a theoretical link between the more or less pragmatic diagnoses of nursing and a general systems model is similar to the recurrent efforts that are made to overcome the narrow scope of individual sciences by means of cross-disciplinary thinking (Grassi & Uexküll, 1951). Here, King reveals the influence of researchers like Bertalanffy, who as professor of theoretical biology and editor of the Yearbook of the Society for General Systems wished to create a cybernetic framework from biology, mathematics, social science, and philosophy to draw an overarching natural philosophy.

Growth and development are linked with the concept of open systems, which, on coming into contact with other systems, undergo continuous, irreversible, and unpredictable change. Feedback mechanisms, whose existence has been demonstrated through the physical observation of nature, and processes in which minor events trigger a complete transformation of a system make a linear causality approach appear far too limited for such a natural philosophy. Building on human knowledge is nevertheless possible through "creative cognition" (Bertalanffy, 1967, p. 91), whereby structures and similarities between phenomena are identified on the basis of probability and correlation theories.

In the 1980s the theoretical foundation used by Bertalanffy underwent further development under the heading "chaos theory" (Briggs & Peat, 1993). Taking up this concept in nursing theory, Rogers formulated her "space-age paradigms" (1991) in which the basic terms of "homeodynamics" are derived from abstract systems. These terms are meant to explain the linkage between the effects of energy fields, patterns, and environments, as well as to make visible the nature of the changes in them. When nurses and caregivers are plagued with doubts by constructivist assertions that there is no such thing as truth, they can now put their hopes once more in an ontological perception of the world order. The "art" of nursing is then, in very general terms, "the utilization of scientific nursing knowledge for the betterment of people" (Rogers, as cited in Fawcett 1995, p. 378). In this approach, which tries to identify complex structures in a deductionist fashion, practical perspectives no longer play any great role, and nurses' training becomes, generally speaking, the "study of unitary, irreducible, individual human and environmental fields: people and their world" (Rogers, 1992, p. 29).

In the current debate on the theory of science, too, models of a new natural philosophy have again become fashionable. Based on the model of the two scientific cultures, fostered by humanities scholars on the one side and by natural scientists on the other, a third culture is emerging (Brockman, 1995). The proponents of the third culture bridge the divisions between the traditional scientific disciplines and uncover the more profound meaning of our lives. At the same time they address the general public in understandable language and are tolerant of different opinions (Brockman, 1995). If a third culture of this kind did indeed assert itself, it would undoubtedly have a great attraction for nursing science. Such a culture through a synthesis of the natural sciences and the humanities may be able to explain in comprehensible terms existential problems of life, meeting the needs of nursing in a large measure. Unfortunately, however, these hopes have been disappointed by all the models that have been put forward, as knowledge becomes generalized, these models constantly fall behind the advances made in the individual disciplines. It is no doubt true that through the specialization and atomization of science general links and relationships frequently remain unrecognized and that an interdisciplinary approach seems essential to ascertain unrecognized general relationships. Nevertheless, the example of the analysis of the phenomena such as health and illness clearly shows that the general view is no substitute for the particular perspective. Although problems connected with changes in people's behavior toward health and illness may often only be solved using an interdisciplinary approach, it is this very shift of perspective between the individual disciplines that enhances our knowledge about these phenomena. When, for example, Luhmann (1990) examines the medical system and its binary coding and comes to the conclusion that, for the doctor's actions, the patient's illness produces the ability to relate (positive value), he is questioning—consciously and necessarily—the self-image of medicine, oriented as it is toward curing the patient. Only a thorough observation and evaluation of the medical (natural science), social (cultural), and psychological (individual) components of behavior can make the significance of health and illness understandable, even though we know full well that every observation has its own perspective as well as its blind spot. Furthermore, these dimensions may be involved to quite different degrees in a concrete situation or behavior so that from the point of view of nursing, too, the demand for a general perspective does not lead us any further.

NURSING SYSTEMS MODELS

Having examined how theories derived from sociology or how systems thinking has been harnessed in nursing science, we return at this point to Parson's original concepts before pursuing other paths of development and without concerning ourselves any further at this stage with a general natural philosophy or its counterpart in nursing theory. In the following, it is intended to examine those approaches that look at systems and subsystems and their relations to environment (that is, nursing models within the "totality paradigm" in the terminology of Parse [1987]).

In her reflections on "nursing and the systems perspective," Neuman (1995, 1997) states that she is guided by Bertalanffy; her notion of holism, however, remains pragmatic because she describes the dynamic freedom of personal development and creativity under conditions of stress adaptation. Like King, she makes use of a systems model with the subsystems of person, group, and society and, like Johnson, she uses a stress model based on that of Selye to explain stimulus and response. Neuman develops a systems model that, in times of growing complexity with regard to relationships within society, is aimed at providing the orientation that is needed in the organization, data processing, and activities of nursing. Although this model is intended to unify various health-related theories

(Neuman, 1995, p. 16), it does not try to place itself metatheoretically above the theories but attempts, instead, to create a foundation for nursing processes. Human beings, whom Neumann regards as "clients" from a nursing point of view, build lines of defense and resistance to ward off or cope with stress. The normal defense line is surrounded by a flexible one and acts as a buffer against stress factors, ensuring that the customary degree of wellness is maintained. "The lines of resistance safeguard the basic structure and facilitate reconstitution toward wellness" (Neuman, 1995, p. 46) and, through the body's natural resistance, for example, keep people physically free from harm and preserve their "integrity." There are five significant variables in this process, comprising the physiological, psychological, developmental, sociocultural, and spiritual dimensions. The system's function is aimed "at achieving a dynamic yet stable interrelationship of spirit, mind, and body of the client in a constantly changing environment and society" (Neuman, 1995, p. 16).

Neuman thus uses key elements of systems sociology and social psychology for her model of nursing, while at the same time attempting to solve a number of problems arising from these approaches. Consequently, she introduces the terms energy flux and development continuum to rid her model of any potentially static character it might possess. The problem of distinguishing between within and without is dealt with by means of a differentiated concept of environment, which includes a created environment in addition to the internal and external components. With the fifth variable, spirituality, which she did not add until 1989, she ascribes a special role to consciousness and expanding consciousness to leave enough scope for the individual organization of the system. She provides practical perspectives of action with the categories of primary, secondary, and tertiary prevention, entrusting carers in the health system with a comprehensive set of tasks from lessening the possibility of a confrontation with stress to readjustment and counselling for the restoration of basic resources. Neuman states that "nursing actions are initiated to best retain, attain, and maintain optimal client health or wellness, using the three preventions as interventions to keep the system stable" (1995, p. 33). Accordingly, the stability of the system is established as the overarching goal of nursing. By means of assessment procedures carers and nurses should ascertain how the internal, external, and created environments affect the system and how energy fluxes, stress factors, and the reaction of the lines of defense and resistance either further or hinder a stable interchange between psyche, spirit, and body. Stability, equated by Neuman with well-being, varies along a continuum from generation of energy (negentropy) to loss of energy and warmth (entropy). As Fawcett

(1995) rightly points out, however, the concept of entropy is usually associated with closed systems and its use in connection with human beings would require further elaboration.

In constructing her model Neuman has drawn up a manual to serve in many practical situations, giving a great deal of guidance for gathering information through the integration of psychological knowledge and enabling an important shift of perspective by linking nursing and prevention. However, she has succeeded in integrating neither nursing interaction nor the changing circumstances because feedback and system growth play only a subordinate role. Moreover, to a very large extent her model dispenses with the concept of equilibrium or "steady state" (Bertalanffy, 1968) within a system and thus lacks an important category for health and illness on which theorists like Johnson have laid much emphasis. One of the strengths of the systemic notion of reality is that one can do away with explanations of linear causality and that the focus on influences in systems and subsystems enables a holistic perception. With the limits of causal explanations for health and illness clearly evident in our present age of complex structures and manifold influences, resorting to the notion of equilibrium makes sense. The significance of the equilibrium of the elements—earth, water, fire, and air—for all forms of life as well as Hippocrates' doctrine of the proper mixture of body fluids are known from antiquity. In Asian cultures, moreover, the equilibrium of hot and cold was often regarded as the basis of good health, while in sub-Saharan Africa importance is often attached to the equilibrium of body, mind, and soul, or managing to live in harmony with the living (family, relatives), the dead (ancestors), and the gods.

Because of its holistic approach the theory of system equilibrium is also of help in nursing in the context of relatives and environment, where it is not a question of changing the prevailing circumstances but of changing the behavior of people in their interaction with each other. In her attempt to make use of systems theory for nursing in the context of family and environment, Friedemann (1995) draws on ideas familiar in family sociology and family therapy, drawing up a model that puts health at the centre of the individual system. Action in the system is aimed at achieving system maintenance, system change, coherence (interplay of subsystems), and individuation (the self). Involved in contact with the environment are the dimensions of regulation/control, stability, growth, and spirituality. Energy flux and the overcoming of anxiety are achieved through the congruence (equilibrium and harmony) of the system. The attempt is made to provide information on the relationship between individuals and other individuals, their families, and their social environment. The knowledge and models used, derived from psychology, have already proved their worth in the support and counselling of families by many clinical psychologists such as Kantor, Riemann, and C. G. Jung. Friedemann regards her model as being in keeping with King's approach to nursing theory and also refers to Fawcett's nursing paradigm, according to which nursing, first, is oriented toward three system planes (individual, group, and environment); second, takes into account the dimensions of stability, control, growth, and spirituality; and, third, deals with the "process which enables or promotes the striving for congruence in the system" (Friedemann, 1995, p. 42). At the same time the attempt is made to find a middle course between changing conditions and changing behavior, which is often referred to in health psychology as "empowerment" (Schwarzer, 1992).

If one distinguishes theories according to the extent of their relevance as suggested by Marriner-Tomey (1994), Friedemann's approach has a more limited scope than those of King and Neuman on account of its concentration on the individual in the family. And yet this approach implies important differentiations: goals of health and nursing actions are not formulated merely with system stability in mind but, rather, a description is given of the concept of system equilibrium as well as the whole system with its subsystems.

Differentiated models with corresponding semantics are essential to observe complex reality, posits Luhmann (1992). Were this approach to be pursued further, however, the processes of the functional differentiation of the subsystems and the self-regulation and self-generation of social systems in nursing would have to be further elucidated for, according to Luhmann, complexity is the key characteristic of modern societies. Reducing complexity would, in certain situations, be a task of nursing if nursing represents a specific functional domain in which actions are related to each other meaningfully. Since Luhmann's model is not an applied science, however, the application of his systems theory to nursing issues is a problem that has yet to be solved—unless one considers his approach, based on the possibility of individual choice, to be of no help and favors, instead, factors of social influence in dealing with health and illness.

In summary, it has been shown that systems theory approaches must be given a very differentiated evaluation with regard to their benefits for nursing science. The concepts used, such as individual, environment, stress and burden, equilibrium and stability or feedback, have undergone further development in recent years and must now be reviewed and revised for nursing science. Practice-oriented models are frequently systems based but mostly have the drawback in that they are oriented to the adaptation of the individual to societal conditions and are unable to integrate the asymmetries of interaction, psychical processes, and changes in relationships. At the same time they often encourage the illusion that there are no limits to the regulative capacity of social processes. Systems approaches could be made greater use of in generating key questions of research because all the systems discussed are well suited to assessing individuals and thus in particular to observing behavior. In drawing up a theory for nursing, however, the significance of systems approaches is often overestimated because, in the attempt to explain the use of holistic knowledge for individual behavior, one loses sight, on the one hand, of the individual perspective that is required (as in the role theory) and oversimplifies, on the other, the knowledge derived from other scientific disciplines. In all the approaches presented the hope of a third scientific culture that unites the natural and social sciences to the satisfaction of both sides under the humanistic perspective of helping and caring can be felt—the search for a unitary theory (Moers, Schaeffer, & Steppe, p. 284). As nursing acquires scientific status, however, a fragmentation into schools of thought will not lead us any further. Orientation toward practice demands first and foremost a pluralist attitude to different theoretical approaches as well as an updating of the theoretical sources in the vast store of interdisciplinary knowledge.

SOCIAL SCIENTIFIC REFLECTIONS ON NURSING

The point of departure for these reflections was the assumption that it is impossible to equate sociological with systems theory perspectives—neither in the social sciences themselves nor in nursing science. Important processes of transformation with regard to nursing in society cannot be adequately explained by systems theory. Which far-reaching theoretical approaches may be taken into consideration, then, to provide a scientific basis for nursing practice?

From the ideas and concepts outlined above it is evident that there is no major theoretical model that can be presented as an alternative. Yet there are important implications to be derived for nursing from the social perspective. Besides the many interesting approaches emerging from public health science (Schaeffer, Moers, Steppe, & Meleis, 1994), which it is not possible to discuss here, important impulses for nursing theory can be culled from other social science discourses. The sociology of life histories is a typical example of analyzing how structural elements and individual biographies are interwoven, the link between the framework of socioeconomic conditions and cohort-specific life histories. Ruth Benedict in the English-speaking world and Martin Kohli in German-speaking countries may be named as outstanding representatives of this scientific field. The life history may be marked by continuity, as is presumed to be the case in many traditional societies, or by discontinuity, as is assumed in the case of modern societies (Friebe, 1996). Problems in the transition from one phase of life to another can lead to ruptures or crises, for instance when biographical age does not concur with personal circumstances. An example of this is a spate of early retirement among the workforce, leading to incongruity between the stage a person has reached in the life cycle and the age group to which the person belongs.

In gerontology and care for the elderly, Matilda Riley has become known for her model of age stratification (Riley, 1979), which describes the structural changes that take place and ascribes key categories to the phases of life—to youth, education; to adulthood, work; and to old age, leisure. Changes in the age structure, rising income, increasing participation in politics and new discourses, have resulted in an age-integrating structure (Riley & Riley, 1992). A number of German gerontologists judge aging to be the expression of a high measure of opportunity for self-development (Baltes & Mittelstraß, 1992). Kohli (1992), on the other hand, observes the diminishing importance of work as a structuring force in society but at the same time sees that dimensions of inequality continue to exist. For women, however, the significance of paid employment has risen on the whole, the daily lives of not only women without children but also those who have completed the family phase being oriented toward the requirements of the labor market. Müller (1989) speaks in this connection of the double role women play in the national economy: In theory equal partners at the workplace but mostly unequal partners in practice, they reproduce patterns of social dominance and, through their added responsibility for work in the home, perpetuate the gender hierarchy. Because women are frequent users of the health system as well as representing the largest group employed in it, changes in the patterns of their life courses are of special significance.

In Parson's systems/sociological analysis, long periods of illness or, even worse, invalidity was considered tantamount to deviant behavior, erring from the state of optimum efficiency, unproductive, and therefore subject to a certain tendency toward uniformity of the life course. As the structuring force of a working society weakens, the importance of other forms of social association, such as social networks, grows. Yet, access to public resources continues to be governed by the availability of financial means and, at the same time, the state is increasingly withdrawing from solidarity contracts on social security arrangements. Modern catchwords such as singularization, the monetarization of social relationships, and a change of course in culture and values characterize this development in which the health and care services are becoming a service industry, differentiated according to the potential of the customer.

The changing panorama of illness puts nursing and care in a context of supply and demand to a certain degree. A possible negative scenario, based on a society that no longer has the financial resources to support an ever increasing ratio of the elderly, sick, and unemployed, is just as wide as a positive vision of the future that combines longer life and more freedom of choice with regard to life planning with a greater quality of life. Changes in health are important elements of the ruptures and transitions in the life course and, here, nursing and care play a special role. It therefore makes sense to take advantage of concepts that represent life events for, on the basis of the biographical approach, these are best suited to comprehending the construction of reality of those involved in the nursing system and working out proposals for change that are appropriate for everyday situations. These are of great advantage, too, in nursing didactics (Kollak & Besendorfer, 1996). The knowledge applied in nursing—as long as it is action-oriented—should not only provide support for people in adapting to life events but also contribute toward changing life situations. The social sciences can assist and support nursing science in building its own knowledge and in redefining nursing practice (Perry & Joliey, 1992), this being a prerequisite of successful professionalization. Here, macro perspectives (systems analyses) and micro perspectives (interaction analyses) ought to be combined.

Nursing theory and practice ought to be coupled above all with regard to methods—basing theories on data, as Glaser and Strauss (1967) formulated it. It is not intended, however, to create competition between quantitative and qualitative social research methods; what is intended is that they should complement each other meaningfully, even if for the analysis of concrete nursing actions there is a preference for qualitative methods. Of great help in this respect is a research process model that provides information on the questions asked and the research perspectives as well as on the methods of data collection, reconstruction, and interpretation. Certain knowledge can be distinguished from mere assumptions by testing validity, and the discourse arising from the research allows the group under investigation as well as the scientific community an opportunity for both self-reflection and the continuation of the research process.

On its way toward professionalization nursing has found it difficult to demarcate its own territory of knowledge and distinguish itself from other professions. A certain degree of emancipation from medical paradigms is to be observed (Botschafter & Steppe, 1994), yet the contours of a separate and independent nursing paradigm remain blurred. Nursing knowledge has scarcely been able to take effect as a catalyst for change in nursing practice. Nursing knowledge is no significant cultural capital, as Bourdieu would say, with a high rate of convertibility to other forms of capital, whether social or economic (Bourdieu, 1993). Nursing knowledge has had an inferior status, just as nursing services have only had small economic worth; the working and training worlds of nurses are gender-specific, merely underlining the gender gap; and nursing activities give no priority to developing the personality or shoring up positive changes in society.

As a result of changes in society, nursing itself is undergoing radical transformation, with catchwords such as the nursing market, nursing services, and the new forms of nursing management underlining these developments. Hospitals and homes for the elderly have changed from being institutions with exalted guiding principles and a social mission to fulfil, becoming organizations with rational, purpose-oriented objectives. In the wake of this development, criteria of success, such as profitability and productivity, have been adopted from free enterprise, and it is these that decide an organization's fate. However, it is quickly becoming clear that the structures and laws governing the provision of health care services are not explicable by means of mechanistic models, for procedures and organization do not follow any objectively predictable pattern, and instead of there being one correct solution to a problem there are often many different solutions competing with each other. It thus appears expedient for nursing management to adapt new methods of organization, which in turn are often marked by systemic thinking.

Lineal concepts of organization leadership regarded management as a body of decision-makers whose actions were based on a special knowledge of the objectively existing world and whose decisions were to be handed down from top to bottom and controlled. The result was the emergence of rigid hierarchies and the organization's large dependence on its leaders. Systemic organization concepts, on the other hand, always view the results produced by an organization as an overall achievement of the whole, whereby the interconnections of the single components and the relationship between system and environment are to be analysed in their competition with each other. Nursing is considered to be a "turbulent field," in which leadership means "acting consciously in networked relationships" (Borsi & Schröck, 1995, p. 171). Nursing groups are also social systems, or a "group as a whole" (Tappen, 1986) whose characteristics are not identical with those of its individual members. Autonomous groups control their work themselves and take part in decision making; thus a good working climate with open communication channels are currently rated highly. This shift of perspective is of great significance for nursing management because hospitals and other health care organizations, which seek an expression of shared values, besides being concerned with the smooth running of their services and their organization culture, are thus moving closer to the ideal of a humane health service.

In the discourse of economics systemic thinking is highly valued. Peter Senge has described it as the "fifth discipline" (Senge, 1990), which first makes possible the necessary flexibility in adapting to the continuous change of society. Just as technical systems consist of components, explains Senge, human systems are based on disciplines. The model could quite easily be applied to nursing management: The first discipline, personal mastery, would correspond to nursing knowledge and nursing abilities; the second, mental models of perceiving the world and of alternative action, are reflected in the discussion on theory and nursing ethic; the third, jointly developing a vision, is familiar in nursing as the discussion on establishing guiding principles; and the fourth, team learning, is frequently taken into account in concepts of group nursing and staff development. Systemic thinking, as a fifth discipline, is something that might be strengthened in nursing management.

It was pointed out earlier in this chapter that a process of rethinking has begun in social scientific discourse, which has already led to the dissolution of the dualism encountered in synchronic and diachronic thinking as well as in systemic and historical perspectives. In the logic of a systemic chain of thought, rethinking in nursing would mean a profound change of attitude in which obstacles hindering the development and realization of ideas as well as unreflected structures of the system are recognized, thus enabling new opportunities for action to be developed creatively. Or must one—now as before—analyze power and inequality in society, identifying how much scope there is for action in nursing on the one hand and which changes are necessary in society on the other? As tempting as the systems theory perspective appears, it has repeatedly been shown that ignoring the historically and culturally anchored contradictions in society allows only one-sided, interest-based changes. The analysis of social conditions and understanding human rationality in acting must be taken into consideration in the development of nursing science, and this goes far beyond the functionalist perspective of systems theory approaches.

REFERENCES

Baltes, P. B., & Mittelstraß, J. (Eds.). (1992). *Zukunft des Alterns und gesellschaftliche Entwicklung*. Berlin, Germany: de Gruyter.

Bertalanffy, L. v. (1967). *Robots, men and minds: Psychology in the modern world.* New York: Braziller.

Bertalanffy, L. v. (1968). *General system theory: foundations, development, applications.* New York: Braziller.

Borsi, G., & Schröck, R. (1995). *Pflegemanagement im Wandel.* Berlin, Germany: Springer.

Botschafter, P., & Steppe, H. (1994). Theorie und Forschungsentwicklung in der Pflege. In D. Schaeffer, M. Moers, & R. Rosenbrock (Eds.), *Public health und Pflege* (p. 72). Berlin, Germany: Sigma WZB.

Briggs, J., & Peat, D. (1993). *Die Entdeckung des Chaos*. München, Germany: Hanser (Translation of *Turbulent mirror: an illustrated guide to chaos theory and the science of wholeness.* New York: Harper & Row).

Brockman, J. (1995). *The third culture.* New York: Simon & Schuster.

Bourdieu, P. (1993). *Soziologische Fragen.* Frankfurt, Germany: Suhrkamp.

Fawcett, J. (1995). *Analysis and evaluation of conceptual models of nursing* (3rd ed.). Philadelphia: Davis.

Friebe, J. (1996). *Altern im Senegal.* Saarbrücken, Germany: Breitenbach.

Friedemann, M. L. (1995). *The framework of systemic organization: A conceptual approach to families and nursing.* Thousand Oaks, CA: Sage.

Friedemann, M. L. (1996). *Familien und umweltbezogene Pflege.* Bern, Germany: Huber Verlag.

Glaser, B., & Strauss, A. (1967). *The discovery of grounded theory: Stratagies for qualitative research.* Chicago: Aldine.

Grassi, E., & Uexküll, T. (1951). *Die Einheit unseres Wirklichkeitsbildes und die Grenzen der Einzelwissenschaften.* Bern, Germany: Francke AG.

Johnson, D. E. (1980). The behavioral system model for nursing. In J. P. Riehl & C. Roy (Eds.), *Conceptual models for nursing practice* (2nd ed., pp. 207–216). New York: Appleton-Century-Crofts.

Kim, H. S. (1989). Theoretical thinking in nursing: Problems and prospects. *Recent Advances in Nursing, 24,* 106–122.

King, I. (1981). *A theory for nursing: systems, concepts, process.* Albany, NY: Delmar.

King, I. (1995). A systems framework for nursing: The theory of goal attainment. In M. A. Frey & C. L. Sieloff (Eds.), *Advancing King's framework and theory of nursing* (pp. 14–32). Thousand Oaks, CA: Sage.

Kohli, M. (1992). Altern in soziologischer Perspektive. In P. B. Baltes & J. Mittelstraß (Eds.), *Zukunft des Alterns und gesellschaftliche Entwicklung* (p. 231). Berlin, Germany: de Gruyter.

Kollak, I., & Besendorfer, A. (1996). Pflege des Menschen mit Herzinfarkt. In *Pflegedidaktik.* Stuttgart, Germany: Thieme.

Korte, H. (Eds.). (1993). *Einführung in die Geschichte der Soziologie.* Opladen, Germany: UTB.

Luhmann, N. (1990). *Soziologische Aufklärung.* Opladen, Germany: Westdeutscher Verlag.

Luhmann, N. (1992). *Beobachtungen der Moderne.* Opladen, Germany: Westdeutscher Verlag.

Marriner-Tomey, A. (1994). *Nursing theorists and their work* (3rd ed.). St. Louis, MO: Mosby.

Moers, M., Schaeffer, D., & Steppe, H. (1997). Pflegetheorien aus den USA—Relevanz für die deutsche Situation. In D. Schaeffer, M. Moers, H. Steppe, & A. Meleis (Eds.), *Pflegetheorien—Beispiele aus den USA.* Bern, Germany: Huber Verlag.

Müller, U. (1989). *Frauensozialkunde—Wandel und Differenzierung von Lebensformen.* Frankfurt, Germany: Campus.

Neuman, B. (1995). *The Neuman System Model* (3rd ed.). Norwalk, CT: Appleton & Lange.

Neuman, B. (1997). Pflege und die Systemperspektive. In D. Schaeffer, M. Moers, H. Steppe, & A. Meleis (Eds.), *Pflegetheorien—Beispiele aus den USA* (p. 197). Bern, Germany: Huber Verlag.

Parse, R. R. (1987). *Nursing science: Major paradigms, theories, and critiques.* Philadelphia: Saunders.

Parsons, T. (1971). *The system of modern societies.* Englewood Cliffs, NJ: Prentice-Hall.

Perry, A., & Joliey, N. (1992). *Nursing: A knowledge base for practice.* London: Arnold.

Riley, M. W. (Ed.). (1979). Life-course perspectives. Aging from birth to death. *AAAS Selected Symposium, 30,* 3–13. Boulder, CO: Westview.

Riley, M., & Riley, J. W. (1992). Individuelles und gesellschaftliches Potential des Alterns. In P. B. Baltes & J. Mittelstraß (Eds.), *Zukunft des Alterns und gesellschaftliche Entwicklung* (p. 437). Berlin, Germany: de Gruyter.

Rogers, M. E. (1991). Space-age paradigm for new frontiers in nursing. In M. E. Parker (Ed.), *Nursing theories in practice* (pp. 105–113). New York: National League for Nursing.

Rogers, M. E. (1992). Nursing science and the space age. *Nursing Science Quarterly, 5,* 27–34.

Schaeffer, D., Moers, M., & Rosenbrock, R. (Eds.). (1994). *Public Health und Pflege.* Berlin, Germany: Ed. Sigma WZB.

Schaeffer, D., Moers, M., Steppe, H., & Meleis, A. (Eds.). (1997). *Pflegetheorien—Beispiele aus den USA.* Bern, Germany: Huber Verlag.

Schwarzer, R. (1992). *Psychologie des Gesundheitsverhaltens.* Göttingen, Germany: Hofgrefe.

Selye, H. (1956). *The stress of life.* New York: McGraw-Hill.
Senge, P. (1990). *The Fifth Discipline.* New York: Doubleday/Currency.
Siegrist, J. (1988). *Medizinische Soziologie.* München, Germany: Urban und Schwarzenberg.
Tappen, R. M. (1986). *Nursing leadership.* Philadelphia: Davis.
Zimbardo, P. G. (1995). *Psychologie.* Berlin, Germany: Springer.

9

Existentialism and Phenomenology in Nursing Theories

Hesook Suzie Kim

Existentialism and phenomenology have provided important influences on the development of nursing knowledge since the early 1980s. However, Paterson and Zderad were the pioneers in nursing who adopted the philosophies of existentialism and phenomenology in their proposal for humanistic nursing and nursology contained in their book published originally in 1976. Their work, premised on the rejection of determinism, positivism, and reductionism, was ahead of its time, as nursing in the 1970s was very much preoccupied with the idea to legitimize the discipline as a science in the traditional positivistic mode. Republication of their 1976 book, *Humanistic Nursing*, in 1988 by National League for Nursing indicates the change in the mood embroiling within the theoretical and empirical sectors of nursing for reexamination of nursing's subject matter and its methodology during the last two decades.

Nursing literature of the last two decades is full of philosophical expositions, theoretical proposals, and research that are based on existentialism, phenomenology, or both. However, philosophical orientations and methodological adoptions in nursing studies are as diverse and disparate as the diversity that exists within both existentialism and phenomenology as general philosophies. Hence, we find in the nursing literature those works identifying Husserl, Heidegger, Merleau-Ponty, and Schutz for providing phenomenological foundation and those citing the existential philosophy of Kierkegaard, Jaspers, Marcel, Nietzsche, and Sartre. The term, existential phenomenology, was introduced in a nursing theory by Parse in 1981. Besides Parse and her colleagues whose works are based on Parse's theory, we are beginning to see specific references to existential phenomenology in nursing literature. For example, Häggman-Laitila (1997) examined health as an individual way of existence from an existential phenomenological perspective, and Jones (1998) examined the application of an existential-phenomenological method of clinical supervision in palliative care nursing. Among the nursing theorists, Margaret Newman (1994) has been revising the assumptions undergirding her theory of "health as expanding consciousness" to align with existential phenomenology in her recent writings.

Existential phenomenology as an ontological focus itself is claimed by various scholars to be based on different philosophical sources. It can be traced to Husserl, Heidegger, Merleau-Ponty, Sartre, Jaspers, and Binswanger. The versions of existential phenomenology coming from these philosophers interweave the tenets of existentialism and phenomenology in various ways and selectively. Hence, it is necessary to examine the ontological features of both existentialism and phenomenology before extricating the major themes in existential phenomenology.

PHENOMENOLOGY AND EXISTENTIALISM

As philosophies, phenomenology and existentialism are modern Continental developments as responses to the philosophical traditions of the time entrenched and threaded with the philosophies of Descartes, Kant, and Hegel. These were the inwardly directed turns addressing ontological questions regarding human consciousness and human existence. These were also developments mostly in Germany and France until the middle of the twentieth century, contrasted with the developments of analytic philosophy, positivism and neopositivism, and pragmatism in England and America.

Phenomenology and existentialism as developed from the nineteenth through the twentieth centuries are also not single, unified philosophies. Leading phenomenologists (such as Husserl, Heidegger, and Merleau-Ponty) and existentialists (Kierkegaard, Nietzsche, Jaspers, Marcel, and Sartre) offer somewhat diverse views regarding human experiences, consciousness, existence, and human lot. The relationship between phenomenology and existentialism is elusive and paradoxical as well. Both philosophies are concerned with the existential content of life; address the role of consciousness as the central to the questions of experience, perception, and existence; and are against quantitative methods and causality-explanations. However, in focusing specifically on human existence some existentialists rejects the appropriateness of applying phenomenological analysis for the study of human existence that are thought to be not objectifiable, whereas phenomenology is concerned not only with human existence but with all phenomena that are consciously constituted. It means that they focus on the ontological questions of existence from different angles: phenomenology is concerned with modes of phenomenal existence, while existentialism focuses on the meaning of human existence. Furthermore, the paradoxical relationship between them is rooted in the apparent opening offered by Husserl for the germination of existentialism, the identity of Heidegger and Merleau-Ponty as both phenomenologists and existentialists, and Sartre's commitment to phenomenology (Barrett, 1962).

In turning to phenomenology, it is necessary to begin the exposition from the phenomenology of Husserl and then review some insights regarding the alternative views advanced by two other leading phenomenologists, Heidegger and Merleau-Ponty. This is important because the phenomenological movement originated with Husserl, who remained committed to both Decartes and Kant, although he moved beyond their doctrines regarding *mathesis universalis* and transcendental philosophy (Natanson, 1966). The major tenets of phenomenology are founded on Husserl's words, "To the things themselves ("*Zu den Sachen selbst*"). This notion is tied to the concept of *things* or phenomena as acts of consciousness, that is, constituted in consciousness. Hence, Husserlian phenomenology encompasses three major ideas: the theory of intentionality, essences (*eidos*) or essential structures of things, and phenomenological method as reduction, all of which are interrelated. Husserl's theory of intentionality is concerned with how things are constituted in the life-world (*lebenswelt*), the ordinary world as shaped within the immediate experiences of each person and constituted through human subjectivity and consciousness. Because it is through consciousness that things come to have meanings or exist as such, human acts are also constituted through consciousness and are experiences of meaning. Thus, for Husserl, "intentionality is seen phenomenologically as foundationally given; it is neither deduced from other elements of consciousness or experience nor postulated from observed elements. Consciousness *is* intentionality . . . " (Natanson, 1966, p. 15). This means that experiences are intentional, and that they are constituted to have meanings as essences or essential structures. The essences (*eidos*) or essential structures of things, acts, and experiences are invariant features constituted through consciousness to them.

The phenomenological method developed by Husserl for phenomenological investigation integrates these two ideas, the theory of intentionality and the concept of essences. Phenomenological method is the mode of investigation for phenomena that exist as consciously constituted affairs. It involves both description and analysis. Spiegelberg (1982) identifies seven features of phenomenological method, only three of which are thought by him to be accepted widely by phenomenological proponents: (a) investigating particular phenomena, (b) investigating general essences, (c) apprehending essential relationships among essences, (d) watching modes of appearing, (e) watching the constitution of phenomena in consciousness, (f) suspending belief in the existence of the phenomena, and (g) interpreting the meaning of phenomena.

This statement suggests that the phenomenological method, as it is understood and developed within the school of phenomenologists, is united by certain basic procedures and premises but is also differentiated in important ways. What is important here is that phenomenology cannot be considered without referring to the phenomenological method because it is both philosophy and science and is rooted in Husserl's epistemological focus.

The key features of phenomenological method as advanced by Husserl are (a) phenomenological reduction, (b) eidetic reduction, and (c) *epoché*. The main idea of phenomenological method is reduction. Reduction to Husserl means "a radical shift in attention from factuality and particularity to essential and universal qualities" (Natanson, 1973, p. 65). The phenomenological reduction focuses on consciousness as the essential feature of constituting the world. The aim of the phenomenological reduction is to understand the world as the intentional correlate of transcendental subjectivity by changing the world into a phenomenon that is known in and by consciousness. To do this, it is necessary to "bracket" and suspend all things, as Husserl put it:

> . . . we set all these theses "out of action", as take no part in them; we direct the glance of apprehension and theoretical inquiry to *pure consciousness in its own absolute Being*. It is this which remains over as the "phenomenological residuum" we were in quest of: remains over, we say, although we have "Suspended" the whole world with all things, living creatures, men, ourselves included. We have literally lost nothing, but have won the whole of Absolute Being, which, properly understood, conceals in itself all transcendences, "constituting" them within itself. (Husserl, 1931, p. 154–155)

The eidetic reduction, on the other hand, focuses on essences. In the eidetic reduction, the investigator must grasp the essences of phenomena—the universal and invariant structures—by peeling away the factual and incidental features that are inherent in variations and attending to essences by means of intuition (*Wesensschau*).

Underwriting these two forms of reduction and the phenomenological method itself is the concept of *epoché*, meaning suspension of judgment. It is the means by which phenomenological description aims to achieve descriptive neutrality and the phenomenological attitude of investigation is attained. Husserl specifies the role of phenomenological *epoché* as follows:

> *We put out of action the general thesis which belongs to the essence of the natural standpoint,* we place in brackets whatever it includes respecting the nature of Being: *this entire natural world therefore* which is continually "there for us," "present to our hand," and will ever remain there, is a "fact-world" of which we continue to be conscious, even though it pleases us to put it in brackets. If I do this, as I am fully free to do, I do *not* then *deny* this "world," as though I were a sophist, I *do not doubt that* it is there as though I were a skeptic; but I use the "phenomenological" *epoché*, which *completely bars* me *from using any judgment that concerns spatio-temporal existence*. (Husserl, 1931, p. 107)

Phenomenology as developed by Husserl (the Husserlian version often termed as transcendental phenomenology in a narrow-sense) has culminated into a philosophical tradition with many variants of significance, among which are Heideggerian hermeneutic phenomenology and Merleau-Ponty's phenomenology of perception as notable influences in nursing.

Heidegger moved away from the Husserlian tenets of phenomenology by focusing on the meaning of Being. Heidegger in his *Sein und Zeit* (*Being and Time*) published in 1927 offers the concept of *Dasein* (being there or being-in-the-world) as the pivotal point for analyzing the meaning of Being. Heidegger rejects Husserl's ideas of transcendental consciousness and his phenomenological reduction as the descriptive and analytic methods for understanding phenomena. Instead, Heidegger turns to interpretation as a way to understand the meaning of Being. Hence, Heidegger's main concern was not the meaning of experiences per se, but the meaning of existence. Heidegger (1962) conceives *Dasein* (being there or Being-in-the-world) for each human existence to come in two possible modes: authentic existence (*eigentliche*) or inauthentic existence (*uneigentliche*), in which authenticity is in taking up of one's existence through one's own choices, whereas inauthenticity is in submitting one's choices to others. In addition, Heidegger (1962) discloses that the basic structures of *Dasein* (Being-in-the-world) are primodial moodness (*Befindlichkeit*), understanding (*Verstehen*), and logos (*Rede*), and that temporality encompassing future, past, and present grounds the Being of human being. Heidegger, hence, reformulated phenomenology as a study of ontology in terms of what exists as it appears, transcending the objective-subjective and real-ideal distinctions.

Merleau-Ponty, a contemporary of Sartre and Simone de Beauvoir and an existentialist, was also the most eminent French phenomenologist. Merleau-Ponty, although greatly influenced by Husserl, rejected Husserl's idea of human consciousness and transcendental ego as the foundation of human experiences. Merleau-Ponty, instead, proposed that perception is the source of knowledge, and that human beings are subjects with bodies that are experienced and experience the phenomenal world through perceptions (Merleau-Ponty, 1962). Hence, human existence in the world is through the lived body's involvement with the world through perception. Unlike Heidegger, Merleau-Ponty affirmed the phenomenological method that focuses on lived-experiences or *Lebenswelt* (life-world) as the sources of knowledge, but doubted the possibility of bracketing as a means to gain complete insight into meanings. Both in Heidegger and Merleau-Ponty, phenomenology is turned toward existentialism, moving away from transcendental ego as the source of all meanings and experiences.

Existentialism, although a twentieth century philosophy, is deeply rooted in two nineteenth century philosophers, Friedrich Nietzsche and Søren Kierkegaard. Existentialism, as a philosophic movement addressing the question of being, is traced by Barrett (1962) to have the central and common thread in recasting the individual's relation to the meaning of religion and religious question and elevating the centrality of human choice in the question of existence. Barrett (1962) identifies the following leading existentialists: Jean-Paul Sartre, Simone de Beauvoir, Albert Camus, and Gabriel Marcel among the French; Karl Jaspers, Martin Heidegger, and Martin Buber as the Germans; Vladmir Solovev, Leon Shestov, and Nikolai Berdyaev from Russia; Miguel de Unamuno and Josè Ortega y Gasset as the Spaniards; and the pragmatist William James as representing the United States. These names, of course, reveal the variant nature of existential thinking, especially in terms of human beings' relationships to religion and God.

In existentialism, the human person is the one, being in the world as a free agent that exists in the present but also is open to a future that is determined by one's own choices and actions. Human beings are becoming of themselves through their choices, choices of ways of life (Kierkegaard, 1959) or choices of actions. Human existence through choices is the reality in which the self is embroiled in the choices and the life is projected.

To existentialists, human choices are not framed within any sort of rational grounds but are open to human freedom, making the choices the responsibility of the self. Hence, humans are open to right or wrong ways of choosing: for Kierkegaard (1959) the choice is among the three levels of existence, the aesthetic, ethical, and religious; for Heidegger (1962) it is the choice between the authentic or inauthentic existence; and for Sartre (1956) the choice leads to an action that is either done with sincerity or with bad faith.

Human existence is thus not only living of oneself with choices but also living of choices that is projected into a future—it thus requires humans to commit themselves to the choices that are made with freedom and accompany self-responsibility. Because human existence is viewed to be situated for each individual and in a concrete, temporally situated context, existentialism opposes objectivism, positivism, and idealism. Existentialism is found to be closely related to phenomenology on two accounts: humans' existential reality is grounded in situation and human beings themselves determine their own existence.

EXISTENTIAL PHENOMENOLOGY

It is difficult to identify clearly the exact nature of existential phenomenology, as this label is attributed to various existentialists and phenomenologists in a rather casual manner in the literature. Sattler (1966) suggests that existential phenomenology as a philosophical orientation for psychology has begun to penetrate the American psychological scene by the 1960s. Sattler (1966) identifies existential phenomenology as an approach that is based on the existential notions about human existence, combined with the phenomenological idea of temporality. He states that the basic thesis of existential phenomenology is: " . . . man is in his inherent nature continually in the process of becoming. In becoming, man also transcends his physical limitations and is not simply a spatiotemporally defined entity. Temporality implies that knowledge of the future is incorporated into man's present action" (Sattler, 1966, pp. 291–292).

More specifically, three versions of existential phenomenology may be identified in association with the philosophical orientations of Sartre, Heidegger, and Merleau-Ponty. Existential phenomenology with a strong identification with Sartre as seen in Gordon's work (1995) is characterized by its commitment to the study of human existence in which human freedom and consciousness projects the self with choices.

Existential phenomenology of Heidegger is based on his notion of *Dasein* as a fundamental ontology by which humans are already involved in an ongoing world. For Heidegger, phenomenology is exactly a study of being, the method of ontology. On the other hand, Merleau-Ponty's existential phenomenology is grounded in his phenomenology of perception and his rejection of transcendental ego.

What is clear from these identifications is that existential phenomenology in general is grounded in the ontology of existentialism and the method of phenomenology. However, the phenomenological method committed by existential phenomenology is not that of Husserl, as existentialists reject the key tenets of Husserl's phenomenology such as *eidos*, transcendental ego, bracketing, meaning constituted by consciousness as well as phenomenological reduction.

PARSE'S THE HUMAN BECOMING THEORY

Parse proposed the Human Becoming Theory in 1981 first as the Man-Living-Health theory, changing its name in 1992 to the current version. Parse claims that her theory is a human science theory with the principal orientation to the concept of "human becoming" as "a unitary construct referring to the human being's living health" (Parse, 1997, p. 32). She particularly specifies that the assumptions of the theory have been constructed by synthesizing the ideas from Rogers' science of unitary human beings and existential phenomenology. Existential phenomenological thoughts are drawn primarily from Heidegger, Sartre, and Merleau-Ponty (Parse, 1997). She also cites Kierkegaard as providing the concept of human subject (Parse, 1981).

She provides nine philosophical assumptions for the theory that resulted from the synthesis of selected ideas from Rogers' science of unitary human beings and existential phenomenology. They are as follows:

1. The human is coexisting while coconstituting rhythmical patterns with the universe.
2. The human is open, freely choosing meaning in situation, bearing responsibility for decisions.
3. The human is unitary continuously coconstituting patterns of relating.
4. The human is transcending multidimensionally with the possibles.
5. Becoming is unitary human living health.
6. Becoming is a rhythmically coconstituting human-universe process.
7. Becoming is the human's patterns of relating value priorities.
8. Becoming is an intersubjective process of transcending with the possibles.
9. Becoming is unitary human evolving (Parse, 1997, p. 32).

Undergirding these philosophical assumptions are two tenets of existential phenomenology, intentionality and human subjectivity; and three principles (resonancy, helicy, and integrality) of Rogers' science. These provide concepts that are directly or indirectly inferred in the philosophical assumptions. The concepts are coconstitution, coexistence, and situated freedom from existential phenomenology, and energy field, openness, pattern and organization, and multidimensionality from Rogers. In addition, from these philosophical assumptions Parse draws three major themes of her theory: meaning, rhythmicity, and cotranscendence, which lead to three principles of the theory as the following:

1. Structuring meaning multidimensionally is cocreating reality through the languaging of valuing and imaging.
2. Cocreating rhythmical patterns of relating is living the paradoxical unity of revealing-concealing, enabling-limiting while connecting-separating.
3. Cotranscending with the possibles is powering unique ways of originating in the process of transforming (Parse, 1981, p. 69).

According to Parse, all nine philosophical assumptions have embedded in them the concepts drawn from existential phenomenology and Rogers. This means that each of the assumptions has ideas from both sources integrated into a unified set. Hence, fundamentally, two distinct but interrelated questions are raised in viewing Parse's theory within the ontological orientation of existential phenomenology: (a) Are the assumptions advanced for the theory coherently and heuristically in alignment with the major tenets of existential phenomenology? and (b) can the ideas drawn from existential phenomenology be articulated with the ideas of Rogers' science of unitary human beings to form the foundation for the Human Becoming Theory?

Parse's articulation of the two tenets (intentionality and human subjectivity) of existential phenomenology comes mostly from Heidegger. She then concludes that these two tenets lead to the assumptions about humans that "man coconstitutes situations with the world, man experiences existence as coexistence, and man has freedom in situation" (Parse, 1981, p. 20). How would existentialists (especially those cited by Parse, such as Heidegger, Merleau-Ponty, and Sartre) interpret co- in coexistence and coconstitution? From Heidegger, at least, *Dasein* is structured existentially by moods (*Befindlichkeit*), understanding (*Verstehen*), and logos (*Rede*), maintaining the self and the world both in diametrical connections and in embeddedness. It appears then the terms starting with co-, when they are used in reference to humans and the universe, also must mean existential structuring of the universe in and with the humans in a side-by-side fashion. This does not seem to align with the ontology of existentialism, as existentialism is a philosophy of human existence, not of universal existence. Hence, for Parse to create the concepts of coexistence and coconstitution to be foundational for her theory, it is necessary for her to develop an ontology that will encompass the co-notion of existence.

The second question is concerned with the appropriateness of articulating the philosophy of existentialism with Rogers' science. The principles and concepts from Rogers' science articulated and retained in the assumptions are openness, human-universe mutual process, rhythmicity, patterning, and multidimensionality. The concept of openness from Rogers refers to the openness of humans and environments in relation to each other and is closely related to the concept of human-universe mutual process. These two concepts in Rogers' science of unitary human beings provide the principles by which human beings and their environments are interpenetrating and moving along together. These are counter to existential phenomenology. The focal point of being in existential phenomenology is the humans who have the subjectivity, are making choices, and are the ones structuring their existence in the world, although not apart and away from the world but not in a mutual sense except with other humans. The concepts of rhythmicity and patterning, although drawn originally from Rogers, have been revised and defined uniquely in Parse's theory. Although these concepts definitionally do not violate the major tenets of existential phenomenology, it is important that the theory does not presuppose the existence of essential types or forms of rhythm and pattern. In addition, the concept of multidimensionality is brought in from Rogers' science and indicates the existential realm that goes beyond the spatiotemporal boundary. It is in line with the thought in existentialism that considers human existence not just as a spatiotemporal one.

This exposition suggests that the articulation of existential phenomenology in Parse's Human Becoming Theory is both illuminating and force-fitting mainly because she tried to reconcile this philosophical foundation with the Rogers' science of unitary human beings. Rogers' unitary human beings coming from the background of holism assumes mutuality of humans and their universe. This foundation puts humans not at the core but at the same plane with the environment (or the universe) in examining human-matters. This is quite different from existential phenomenology's centering of humans and human existence. This seems to be the irreconcilable, fundamental contradiction between the two foundations said to be the major sources for providing philosophical assumptions of Parse's theory.

CONCLUSIONS

The foregoing exposition provides the background for considering existentialism and phenomenology as a possible ontological focus for nursing theories. To take existentialism or phenomenology as an ontological focus for a nursing theory, it is necessary to pose the following questions:

- What is the meaning of human health within the tenets of existentialism or phenomenology?
- How is the experience of human health and health care interpreted in terms of human subjectivity, freedom of choice, existential meaning, temporality, situatedness, and historicity?
- What is the meaning of human health existentially or phenomenologically?
- What does it mean to be in human practice existentially or phenomenologically?
- How is the role of researcher (investigator) articulated for existential or phenomenological knowledge of human health, suffering, and practice?
- How is it possible to distinguish existential or phenomenological researcher from existential or phenomenological practitioner?

Theories emerging from such foundations must assume a different format from those theories based on other ontological foci, which permit explanation or prediction. Basically, theories with the ontological focus of existentialism or phenomenology will need to be oriented either to the specification of methodology or the descriptive features regarding the realm of human life such as human health.

REFERENCES

Barrett, W. (1962). *Irrational man: A study in existential philosophy.* Garden City, NY: Doubleday Anchor.

Gordon, L. (1995). *Bad faith and antiblack racism.* Atlantic Highlands, NJ: Humanities Press.

Häggman-Laitila, A. (1997). Health as an individual's way of existence. *Journal of Advanced Nursing, 25,* 45–53.

Heidegger, M. (1962). *Being and time* (J. Macquarrie & F. Robinson, Trans.). New York: Harper & Row. (Original work published 1927)

Husserl, E. (1931). *Ideas: General introduction to pure phenomenology* (W. R. B. Gibson, Trans.). New York: Macmillan. (Original work published 1913)

Jones, A. (1998). "Out of the sighs"—an existential-phenomenological method of clinical supervision: the contribution to palliative care. *Journal of Advanced Nursing, 27,* 905–913.

Kierkegaard, S. (1959). *Either/or, Vols. I & II* (D. F. Swenson & L. M. Swenson, Trans.). Princeton, NJ: Princeton University Press. (Original work published in 1843.)

Merleau-Ponty, M. (1962). *Phenomenology of perception* (C. Smith, Trans.). London: Routledge & Kegan Paul (Original work published 1945)

Natanson, M. (1966). Introduction. In M. Natanson (Ed.), *Essays in phenomenology* (pp. 1–22). The Hague, Netherlands: Martinus Nijhoff.

Natanson, M. (1973). *Edmund Husserl: Philosopher of infinite tasks.* Evanston, IL: Northwestern University Press.

Newman, M. (1994). *Health as expanding consciousness.* New York: National League for Nursing.

Parse, R. R. (1981). *Man-living-health: A theory of nursing.* New York: Wiley.

Parse, R. R. (1992). Human becoming: Parse's theory of nursing. *Nursing Science Quarterly, 5,* 35–42.

Parse, R. R. (1997). The human becoming theory: The was, is, and will be. *Nursing Science Quarterly, 10,* 32–38.

Patterson, J. G., & Zderad, L. T. (1976). *Humanistic nursing.* New York: Wiley.

Patterson, J. G., & Zderad, L. T. (1988). *Humanistic nursing* (2nd ed.). New York: National League for Nursing.

Sartre, J. (1956). *Being and nothingness,* Special abridged edition (H. E. Barnes, Trans.). Secaucus, NJ: The Citadel Press. (Original work published in 1943.)

Sattler, J. M. (1966). The existential-phenomenological movement and its impact on contemporary American psychology. *Journal of Existentialism, 6,* 289–294.

Spiegelberg, H. (1982). *The phenomenological movement: A historical introduction* (3rd ed.). The Hague, Netherlands: Martinus Nijhoff.

10

Humanism in Nursing Theory: A Focus on Caring

May Solveig Fagermoen

The philosophies of humanism and caring have been fundamental to nursing throughout its history, shaping the basic character of nursing, namely, that nursing inherently is a moral practice. Viewed as a service to humankind, nursing throughout has been guided by a moral motivation to act in the best interest for those in need of nursing care.

In modern nursing, Florence Nightingale, a true humanist, stands out as a warrior in her fight for patients' dignity and decent care, first during the Crimean war and later when she worked to better nursing care and the conditions within hospitals. In her view, caring for patients implied providing the best possible environment to allow natural processes of healing to take place and to help patients meet their physical needs in an individualized manner. Both action orientations were to be based on astute observations and knowledge. From this perspective several theorists have developed further her ideas of what nursing is all about, what constitutes good nursing care, and how to think and act to provide the best possible care within a humanistic tradition. For example, Abdellah, Henderson, and Orem further our understanding of nursing as a complementary assistance toward fulfilling patients' basic needs when they are lacking the knowledge, strength, or will to carry out the necessary activities themselves and in a manner in which the patients' independence and self-care are upheld and restored. Other theorists, such as Peplau, Travelbee, and Watson, have developed further the ideas about individualized care, specifically in relation to the interpersonal domain of nursing, while Leininger, with her concept of transcultural care, has extended our vision of what nursing care is all about.

To understand their theoretical perspective in advancing nursing, it is useful to examine their fundamental ideas. A basic building block in these as well as other nurse-theorists' works is the idea of humanism. Therefore, in this chapter humanism will be traced from a historical perspective, how it is developed within other disciplines, how it has influenced nursing's disciplinary culture, and finally, Watson's theory of human care will be viewed within this general frame. The chapter will conclude with what humanism and caring means for nursing practice and advancement of nursing knowledge.

HUMANISM: TRACING THE DEVELOPMENT

Today, the word *humanism* has many connotations. Generally, humanism is understood as the tendency to emphasize humans and their status, importance, powers, achievements, or authority. Humanism is also referred to as a school of thought, as a philosophical movement, and a worldview, which assign human beings a special position in the world at large. In the literature different strands of humanism are distinguished by descriptive adjectives such as religious humanism, secular humanism, Renaissance humanism, Enlightenment humanism, and so forth. This reflects that humanism as we understand it today has been a movement over time, molded by a theological or atheistic worldview in different historic contexts. The common ontological characteristics across different denominations are the centrality of man, his powers, and potentialities. This presentation of humanism is not aimed at covering every aspect of humanism in philosophic writings but to select and include those ideas, which to my knowledge have had the greatest impact on the development of nursing science.

Although the word humanism came into usage at a later time, the movement or philosophical idea of humanism was rediscovered in Italy in the second half of the fourteenth century at the advent of the Renaissance. Thinkers in this period sought to reintegrate humans into the world of nature and history and to interpret them in this perspective. This movement was the renaissance of antiquity, "the preservation and cultivation of the ideals and culture in the classical world" (Luik, 1991a, p. 17). Through the study of the classical literature and art, the rebirth of a spirit that humans had possessed in that age and had lost in the Middle Ages could be realized. It denoted a move away from God to humans as the center of interest, which allowed for "a spirit of freedom that provided justification for man's claim of rational autonomy, allowing him to see himself involved in nature and history and capable of making them his realm" (Abbagnano, 1972, p. 70).

The central theme of humanism was the potentialities of humans, their creative powers. These powers, including the power to mold oneself, were latent, to be brought out, and the means to that end was education. The humanists saw education as the process by which humans were lifted out of their natural condition to discover their *humanitas* (humanness). At the end of the fifteenth century *umanista* (humanist) was used to describe the teacher of the classical languages and literatures, as a contrast to *legista*, the teacher of law (Kolenda, 1995). The Renaissance term for what they studied was *Studia humanitatis*, which meant grammar, rhetoric, poetry, history, languages, politics, and moral philosophy. Accordingly, there is the root of the fields of study that today are known as the humanities.

The privilege accorded to the humanities was founded on the conviction that these disciplines alone could educate humans and put them in the position to effectively exercise their freedom. Andic (1991) summarizes the mood of the Renaissance era:

> We need to understand and realize ourselves in our humanity and to cultivate those humane virtues that makes us fully human beings—then where better place to begin this self-study than with the . . . [writings] from outstanding men and women drawn from the treasury of Latin and Greek history and literature, in order to learn by imitating their deeds and avoiding their failures to become such as they are? (p. 90)

God still remained a creator and supreme authority, but His activities were seen as less immediate, more as a general control than as a day-to-day interference. This change in belief combined with an emphasis on humans' powers of reason, encouraged their ability to find out about the universe by their own efforts, and more and more to control it. Hence, this worldview enabled a scientific outlook to arise that saw the universe as governed by general laws, albeit these were laid down by God.

> When the fourteenth and fifteenth century humanists and philosophers said that man is placed in the center of the world and can become what he himself chooses, they did not mean that everything is permitted to him; they said that he is the middle, not as the *measure* of all things but as the *mediator* of the divine vision and love. . . . They thought that God is fully divine only in man. (Andic, 1991, pp. 92–93)

The breach between art and science had not yet taken place. Humans, seen as natural beings whose interests are to make nature their domain, were given tools, their senses, through which they could question and understand nature. Humanity with all its facets and distinct capabilities, problems, and possibilities was examined in paintings and poetry. The great artists of this time, Michelangelo and Leonardo da Vinci, who both also studied anatomy and physiology, rediscovered the human body through drawings and paintings. Bullock (1985) made this comment, "The combination of the observation, description and representation of nature has been claimed as one of the indispensable prerequisites for the burst of scientific innovation which begins with the humanist-scientist Galileo" (p. 39). Hence, Renaissance humanism is generally considered to be one of the conditions that contributed to the birth of modern science.

In Renaissance humanism, the insistence on the value and centrality of human experience was reflected in the core idea, that of "*dignitas*—the proper relationship between God and nature" (Madigan, 1991, p. 327). This Renaissance concept—the dignity of man—reflects a confidence in the value of humans and their work and is grounded in the latent power women and men possess. The ability to create and communicate in language, the arts, and institutions and also to observe themselves, to speculate, imagine, and reason " . . . enable men and women to exercise a degree of freedom of choice and will, to change course, to innovate and thus to open the possibility . . . of improving themselves and the human lot" (Bullock, 1985, p. 156). The concept of human dignity was recovered and restated later, as in the Enlightenment, when human dignity no longer was seen as linked to humans' divine origin, but to their rational possibilities in this world. The concept of human dignity and that which it implies is the foundation for human rights as we know them today.

Humanism in the Enlightenment is linked to the eighteenth-century thinkers "who believed that the central concern of human existence was not the discovery of God's will, but the shaping of human life and society according to a set of universally acknowledged rational principles" (Luik, 1991b, p. 118). The Enlightenment humanists' enormous confidence in and commitment to human reason was reflected in their belief in the centrality of science and the scientific method. One of the great philosophers at that time, Kant (1724–1804) claimed that "Enlightenment is man's emergence from his self-concurred immaturity," with the "motto of enlightenment therefore: *Sapere aude!* Have the courage to use your *own* understanding!" (cited in Luik, 1991b, p. 119).

Reason was not only the discovery of facts, but also a base from which one partly could create moral principles, that is, giving a grounding for morality. Two foundational principles in Kant's ethics are still recognized today: (a) persons as ends in themselves, all rational beings exist as an end in themselves and not merely as means to be arbitrarily used by this or that will, and (b) the centrality of freedom, only human persons can freely set and achieve ends, and the unique value of human persons is to be found in their self-determining ends. Enlightenment humanism may be defined by the confidence in human autonomy, "an autonomy secured through the creative and ordering power of reason" (Luik, 1991b, p. 118). Among others, Hume (1711–1776) was a strong opponent to Kant in regard to the grounding of morality in reason. He did not reject that reasoning is important in morality, but the primacy of rationality. According to Baier (1987), he held that "morality rests ultimately on sentiment, on a special motivating feeling . . . our capacity for sympathy with other's feelings" (p. 41). The interdependence between persons requires collaboration and accordingly, for Hume, morality depends on "a *reflective* sentiment, and on self-corrected self-interest and corrected sympathy" (Baier, 1987, p. 47). Hume's thoughts on morality are relevant today in view of the increased emphasis on relational ethics and the ethics of caring.

As in the Renaissance era, individual freedom was a central value, in addition to the values of equality and tolerance, which were emphasized and reflected in their beliefs in the moral sense of responsibility and the possibility of progress. Although the Enlightenment humanists believed in the primacy of reason, it was to be used in the service of social and political reform. These characteristics were later revived in pragmatism, which was the most influential philosophy in America in the first quarter of the twentieth century. Humanism in pragmatism will be addressed later in the chapter.

The belief in the centrality of science, its method and orderly explanations, formulated in propositions and laws proliferated in the next centuries and expanded into all aspects of human life. Darwinism was a major force that stimulated the extension of scientific explanations beyond the natural sciences to social sciences. It is also first with Darwinism that humanism acquired its modern association with atheism and agnosticism. Dilthey (1833–1911), a German philosopher, was one of the first to criticize this single-science conception and opposed the strategy of applying the scientific method on human phenomena other than the natural ones because it was inappropriate: such phenomena required different methods. Hence, humans' unique position in the world of nature was reemphasized.

Dilthey did not believe that human life could be understood by using the explanatory model that classifies events according to the laws of nature (Nerheim, 1995). Human life is lived in a cultural world created by human beings. This, a shared world of ideas, values, beliefs, languages, symbols, and institutions, can accordingly be grasped and understood from the inside, as humans we can enter into them. This conception of the common ground is basic to the introduction of hermeneutics in the social sciences. Dilthey argued: the methods needed to uncover these phenomena, which constitute an inner world of purpose and meaning, have to be of an interpretative nature and cannot be revealed by the methods of natural sciences (Skirbrekk & Gilje, 1987).

Purpose and meaning cannot be explained, only understood, and understanding (*Verstehen*) requires a common ground, that is, human beings can understand what human beings have created. Understanding in this context is conceived as a mental act, it is an activity, not merely an experience. Hence, Dilthey insisted on a difference between explanation and understanding, the first can be sought by the scientific methods, the latter by the hermeneutic method. This general method of comprehension of meaning is central to the *Geisteswissenschaften* (translated as *human sciences* in America, see Polkinghorne (1983, pp. 283–289) for a clarification on the choice of English words). However, Dilthey did not see the hermeneutic method as the only and exclusive method in the human sciences. Humans are not only pure *Geist* (spirit), therefore other methods may be needed: it is the topic at hand that decides the choice of method (Skirbrekk & Gilje, 1987). Thus, the human sciences must conceive of humans as both subject and object. As subject humans must be understood as creators of their own world and as beings controlling their actions, humans are creative, strive for meaning, and act intentionally. Understanding humans as object, their actions can be conceived in causal terms, however, there are limits to causal explanations because humans are creative beings and can change. Thus, Dilthey underscored the relativistic nature of humans and human life; everything is dependent on time and place.

In contrast to Dilthey's exposition of hermeneutics as a method central to the Geisteswissenschaften, Heidegger (1889–1976) considered hermeneutics primarily as a process fundamental to human life, that is, his position is ontological. Heidegger argued that understanding (*Verstehen*) is a basic form of human existence, it is not the way we know the world, it is the way we are. To be human is to be interpretative; humans are hermeneutic beings whose whole lives are forever interpretation. Hence, Heidegger saw hermeneutics as the basic pattern of human understanding: we vacillate between the known and the unknown, between the parts and the whole, continuously seeing new sides, gaining new insights, possibly seeing better and more true, but always as imperfect humans in our search (Skirbrekk & Gilje, 1987). Hence, the act of interpretation is linked with being, "interpretation is the activity that enables us to experience the world . . . everything that exists in the world exists for people through the act of interpretation and understanding" (Thompson, 1990, p. 237). This distinction between hermeneutics based in ontology and hermeneutics discussed from an epistemological position (as Dilthey) is important, although not always recognized. Thompson (1990) named these as two of the "three conversations in hermeneutics"; the third being the methodological discussion that voices questions about the proper methods for data-collection and analysis in an interpretative study.

In his philosophical analyses, Heidegger sought answers to the overriding question of the meaning of being (Nicolaisen, 1997). In his major work, *Being and Time,* he argued that the answer to what makes reality meaningful must be sought from the perspective of what is particular to the being of man, his being in the world. One result of this analysis was discussed above, humans' living as being a continuous interpretative process. Foundational to this answer is Heidegger's position that meaning is not something created by ideas, but is evolving as we involve ourselves in the world. Humans' are relational beings, from the moment of birth, thrown into the world; humans are in relation to other beings and other things. Humans are not conceivable without relationships. The concept *Sorge*, (translated to *care/caring* in English), is used by Heidegger to characterize the basic principle of humans' being. This being is constituted as a being-in-the-world and as a being-together-with-others (Nerheim, 1995).

Hence, our being presupposes the being of others. Our existence is communion: our foundational characteristic is that we are living because of and for the others for our own sake. The consideration and care for others in their interest are in our own interest. "Our task in this world is one: we are and have to be" (Nicolaisen, 1997, p. 529). This is man's freedom, to choose whom to be. Further, human's interpretative nature is a premise for the comprehension of (a) what is in the other's interest and (b) seen from the other's perspective. However, for care to be authentic, the presence of an attitude (*Befindlichkeit*) in which one acknowledges the other's personhood is required. The concept of *Sorge* emphasizes that authentic self-understanding can only be found by relating to the world through practical work and at the end, the answer to whom you are has reference to the world in which you live and act, the human life-world (Nerheim, 1995, p. 291).

Heidegger was a critic of the humanisms of the past, which he saw as resting on the notion that the dignity of humans was tied to the assumption that humans are the rational animals (Goicoechea, Luik, & Madigan, 1991). He posited that for humans to live in their highest dignity it is not enough for them to think of themselves as rational animals and argued for a return to "original humanism which [he] refers to as 'emediating and caring, that man be human and not inhuman, that is, outside his essence' " (cited in Goicoechea, 1991, p. 21). In this we see traces of Hume's standpoint in regard to the foundation of morality.

In North America, humanism is clearly reflected in and developed further in the philosophical movement of pragmatism, which emerged toward the end of the nineteenth century. This movement, which is foremost linked to the ideas of Charles S. Pierce (1839–1914), William James (1842–1910), and John Dewey (1859–1952), "is best understood as in part, a critical rejection of much traditional academic philosophy and, in part, a concern to establish certain positive aims" (Thayer, 1972, p. 430). Pragmatism sought to reconcile incompatibilities between philosophical idealism and realism, that is, it was struggling with the questions: does reality exist only in human experience and given in the form of perceptions and ideas or does reality exist in the form of essences or absolutes that are independent of human experience? (Maines, 1992).

According to Francis (1991), the basic pragmatist thought is:

> There exist no permanent essences of any kind, including none of humankind. Everything is in a constant reorganization by interacting and transacting with something. . . . Basically all that exists is change, and the interactions and complexity or diversity of change . . . human existence, life, and all experience, including the intellectual, are contingent, tentative, developing aspects of change. (pp. 238–239)

Hence, such dualisms as matter and mind, object and subject, reality and thought collapse (Diggins, 1994).

Strongly influenced by the evolutionary theory of Darwin, pragmatists focused on human beings' struggles for existence in an ever-changing world in which they themselves are changing, individually and socially. *Experience* is a fundamental term in pragmatism and conceived as "an active, interacting, undergoing, undertaking, and reconstructing of life's events" (Francis, 1991, p. 236). Hence, humans' capacity for problem-solving is central to the pragmatic school of thought. Rather than being passive responders to stimuli, humans are active, creative organisms, empowered with agency. The human being is embedded in an on-going complex nature and is engaged continuously in learning-by-doing, to make sense of things, or to solve problems. Hence, human life "is [seen] as a dialectical process of continuity and discontinuity and therefore [as] inherently emergent" (Maines, 1992, p. 1532). In an interactive relationship, humans and society are constantly shaping and reshaping themselves, sustained by symbolic communication and language. In the pragmatic school of thought, this interdependence between the individual and the society included also the individual's responsibility for social reform and moral conduct for the public good. The pragmatic method, synonymous with the method of science, was hailed as supreme to solve problems of both social and moral character, as expressed by Dewey (1976/1916).

> Social questions are capable of being intelligently coped with only to the degree in which we employ the method of collected data, forming hypotheses, and testing them in action which is characteristic of natural science, and in the degree in which we utilize in the behalf of the promotion of social welfare the technical knowledge ascertained by physics and chemistry (p. 343). . . . The social interest, identical in its deepest meaning with a moral interest, is necessarily supreme with man. (p. 345)

Pragmatism represented also a critique of society, and both Dewey and Mead, together with other pragmatists, engaged themselves in programs for social change in Chicago.

The basic principle of pragmatism whose Greek root word (*pragma*) means action, is that "ideas must be related to practical consequences and must be responsive to the broader problems of civilization" (Kurtz, 1972, p. 88). Education was seen as synonymous with democracy, providing liberation from oppressive authorities. In education and social life generally, the pragmatic principle was the ideal, that is, all ideas should be submitted to a threefold procedure: cooperative inquiry, experimental testing, and judgment arrived at through public consensus. Mead (1964a) outlined the procedure of a discourse ethics based on the same principle.

Hence, pragmatist thoughts can be seen as roots to diverse movements of today, such as, problem-based learning, Habermas' critical theory, and the corresponding action research. The philosophical movement of pragmatism has been influential in many fields, especially in education, psychology, and sociology. Many of the theories adapted into nursing can be traced to pragmatism, such as Mead's thoughts reflected in symbolic interactionism and Glaser and Strauss' Grounded theory, Dewey's educational theory, and humanistic psychology.

HUMANISM REFLECTED IN PSYCHOLOGY AND SOCIOLOGY

As outlined earlier, a basic humanistic thought in pragmatism is the linkage between humans' self-generating powers and social reorganization. While both concepts were developed further within American sociology and social psychology, the founders of humanistic psychology adopted primarily the former concept in their shared view that a person is a "being-in-the process-of-becoming." DeCarvalho (1991, pp. 83–84) summarized their views in this manner:

> Each human being . . . is a unique organism with the ability to direct and change the guiding motives or "project" of life's course. In the process of becoming, one must assume the ultimate responsibility for the individualization and actualization of one's existence. To reach the highest levels through the process of becoming, a person must be fully functioning (Rogers) or functionally autonomous (Allport); the self must be spontaneously integrated and actualizing (Maslow); there must be a sense of self awareness, centeredness (May), and authenticity of being (Bugental). (pp. 83–84)

The view of the person as being in a process of becoming was these psychologists' attack on and answers to the dominant psychology at that time, behaviorism. Thus, the reflection of the pragmatists' emphasis on humans as being active and creative, shaping their world, and not being passive and mere responders to stimuli, is evident. These psychologists also introduced phenomenology and existentialism into a traditional positivist milieu. In this, one can see the influence of the pragmatist philosopher James, who according to Diggins (1994) "gave philosophical legitimacy to all kinds of experience, personal and spiritual as well as physical and factual . . . making room for the subjective as well as the objective, [he] paved the way for making American philosophy receptive . . . to existentialism and phenomenology" (p. 126). An American psychologist often referred to in nursing, Amadeo Giorgi (1970), is also based in phenomenology and existentialism. He was the first to argue that psychology ought to be understood as a "human science" considering its subject matter: the person-in-becoming. His position was taken also as a reaction against behaviorism and its ideal of natural science as the proper and only method of psychological research (Polkinghorne, 1983). Giorgi has developed his own method for phenomenological study, which is frequently used and referred to by nurse researchers.

As seen, in psychology the tension between experimental and experiential paradigms of understanding human nature was introduced just after the World War II. These paradigms, as discussed by Dilthey 100 years earlier, refer to the contrast between explanation and understanding as the goal of scientific work. This has also been an issue of discussion in the social sciences (Fay & Moon, 1994) and in medicine (Schwartz &

Wiggins, 1985). The former argued the benefit of and need for both in furthering knowledge development in their fields while the latter called for a humanistic approach in medicine, "Without humanism of medicine we remain blind to the complexities and details of the human evidence. . . . Only this enlarged understanding of the humanness and individuality of patients can provide the evidential context for a medical science of health and illness" (p. 359). In nursing, humanism has a long tradition, however, only from the late 1970s is there growing evidence for its impact on methodology in nursing research.

Two of the early theorists in pragmatism, Cooley (1864–1929) and Mead (1863–1931), explicated further the ideas of humans' self-generative powers and social reorganization. Both rejected the dualism between mind and society and developed theories about the interdependence between the two. Their theories have had profound influence in social psychology and sociology in regard to the understanding and studies of roles, social groups, conflicts, negotiations, and organizations, for example, as reflected in the work of Erving Goffman, Anselm Strauss, and Herbert Blumer. Concepts such as *the looking-glass self* (Cooley), and *I* and *Me* and *role-taking* (Mead), are foundational to other theories in sociology, especially within interactionism. The looking-glass self refers to Cooley's theory on the development of self-concepts, that these are behaviorally derived through reflected appraisals of the actions of others in which the primary groups are especially important as they link the person to society. Society, on the other hand, "is an interweaving and interworking of mental selves" (Maines, 1992, p. 1533).

Mead held that mind and selves developed in the social act as humans, through imaginatively placing oneself in the position of others, taking the role of the other, is learning the symbolic meanings embedded in society. This involves "a conflation of subjective and objective processes through which persons adjustively contend with the facts of their environments and simultaneously create new situations" (Maines, 1992, p. 1533). Hence, Mead in his analysis of role-taking, the construction of shared meanings, was concerned with that of "intersubjectivity," a core concept within phenomenology and later discussed and developed further by the sociologist Alfred Schutz (Turner, 1986). Mead explored the concepts of subjectivity and objectivity, represented in the terms I and Me, also in regard to the methods of science (Mead, 1964b). Thus, Mead laid the base for the development of a research method in which both subjectivity and objectivity are combined rather than competing, namely that of grounded theory (Glaser & Strauss, 1967).

When reviewing the names of theorists in both psychology and sociology whose thoughts are rooted in pragmatism and humanism, most can be recognized as central to the development of nursing as a discipline, especially in North America. The founders of humanistic psychology have had great impact on all writings on the interpersonal relationship between nurses and patients, such as those of Travelbee, Peplau, Orlando, Zderad and Paterson, and Watson, who also refers to Giorgi, the phenomenological psychologist. Giorgi is frequently mentioned when research methods within the qualitative paradigm is discussed or outlined in the nursing literature. Interactionism in sociology has had impact on nursing through its theories of socialization, role development, organizational issues, and also through the grounded theory approach in research. One may conclude that humanism and pragmatism are at the center of modern nursing.

HUMANISM OF TODAY

In a recent publication in which the ideas of philosophers from Antiquity to the present time were explored in view of traces of humanism in their thoughts, a critical remark was made: to consider everyone humanists "who are interested in the best life of human beings" is not a useful definition of humanism (Goicoechea, Luik, & Madigan, 1991, p. 36). What then can be said of humanism of today?

In general, humanism is not considered to be one philosophical system but rather a continuing debate in which many different views on humans' place in the order of things and humans' being in the world are the central issues. Several sources reviewed for this chapter argue that a central tenet of humanism is "to acknowledge the humanity in everyone, the capacity of every person to think and act of himself" (Andic, 1991, p. 36). Further, humanism is most often contrasted with other competing positions, such as the supernatural, transcendent position, which consider humanity to be radically dependent on divine order, and the scientific position, which treats humanity scientifically as part of the natural order, on a par with other living organisms. In this cleavage, humanism is placed as a middle position as it discerns in human beings unique capabilities and abilities to be cultivated and celebrated for their own sake. Humanism focuses on humans and the human experience.

> That does not rule out either religious belief in a divine order or the scientific investigation of man as part of the natural order but it makes the point that, like every other belief—including the values we live by, and indeed all

our knowledge—they are derived by human minds from human experience. (Bullock, 1985, p. 155)

Accordingly, humanism accepts that there is more than one way to truth.

Another characteristic of humanism of today is the contrasts between theological and secular underpinnings of the basic values expressed in humanism. One overriding value in humanism is that of human dignity, which from the theological position is founded in the belief that humans are created by God and in God's image, while from a secular position this value is held high because of humans' unique capabilities, particularly their ability to reason, as expressed by Protagoras "man is the measure of all things." Similarly, the value of individual freedom is from a secular position arising from humans' reasoning power, in contrast to the theological belief that freedom is based in a free will given by God. Equality and tolerance are two other values held high in humanism, which may be seen as values derived from human dignity. Hence, these values are given different grounding from these two types of humanism. Both values underscore the interdependence between human beings. This is the foundation for a moral sense of responsibility, and is an impetus for social and political engagement to better the world of humans. Social reconstruction is a central concept in humanism as well as self-realization. Central to these concepts is education, which is seen as a cornerstone for social change. Education is aimed at awakening the possibilities, drawing out the humanness and the all-around development of the personality and the full range of individual talents.

CARING AS THE PHILOSOPHICAL FOCUS

Caring as a phenomenon is as old as humankind. There has always been someone within the family or close social network who was given the responsibility to take care of those not able to do so themselves. To take care of one's own was a duty, others were left to the care of themselves. When presenting caring as a philosophical focus it seems reasonable to start with the advent of Christianity. Christ emphasized, both in his own acts and in his teachings, the need for and importance of caring for those who were sick, weak, fallen, or outcasts regardless of family or social ties. A great contrast to the common practice in the community, Christ's primary commandment "to love thy neighbor as thyself" was a provocation as well as his story of the good Samaritan. These became the ideals of his followers, on which they developed a system of service for those in need, later established as cloisters. Nursing as a social service was, until the Renaissance era, closely associated with these institutions and carried out by nuns.

The Renaissance period, in reintroducing humanism with its emphasis on the unique powers of humans, was the period that also introduced the downfall of the Catholic Church and its power over minds and people. Some of the consequences were that in many places the hospitals of the Church were closed, the sick and helpless were left to their own care, and the ideal of the individual's responsibility for the weak, the sick, and so forth was generally weakened. Institutional care turned into low-grade work for uneducated women, and the quality of care was at a minimum. Generally, this was the situation when modern nursing saw the light with the founding of a nursing school at Kaiserswerth in Germany in 1836 and later through Florence Nightingale's work in the Crimean War and the establishment of her nursing school at St. Thomas Hospital in London.

The caring philosophy of Florence Nightingale evolved from her Christian beliefs and materialized in hands-on-care, first for the soldiers in the Crimean War and later for the most unfortunate in London. Her war was a war on behalf of the sick to make their conditions better. Nightingale's theory on nursing published in *Notes on Nursing* (1860/1969) reflects a caring philosophy in which caring for the patient implies attending to basic needs individually through careful and considerate nursing "to put the patient in the best condition for nature to act upon him" (p. 75). She saw patients' experience of discomfort and suffering to be related to inadequacies in the environment, being it physical (stale air, dirty linen, etc.) or the nurse herself (noise of shoes, loud talk, etc.). Her focus of care was essentially actional not interactional, and the action-orientation was toward the environment: to provide the proper use of warmth, light, air, cleanliness, quiet, and administration of a sufficient and useful diet at the least energy expense for the patient. Thus, to Nightingale caring implied a moral imperative in nursing, realized in actions that assisted the reparative processes in patients and decreased suffering.

Since the emergence of modern nursing, care has been at the core of this service. The centrality of the concepts of care and caring are evident in the vast amount of literature on these subjects. The elaboration on these concepts in the nursing literature, however, is diversified and lacks conceptual clarity. For example, caring is discussed as a generic value; as a trait or an attitude of the nurse; as a characteristic of the nurse-patient relationship; as an intervention; and as philosophy or an ethic of nursing

(Morse, Bottorff, Neander, & Solberg, 1991; Morse, Solberg, Neander, Bottorff, & Johnson, 1990).

Earlier in this chapter, several sources have been referred to who see care as fundamental to human life and as such they have addressed the philosophy of caring. To Heidegger, his concept Sorge (care/caring) characterizes the basic principle of humans' being, that is, care/caring is fundamental to human life; being-in-the world and being-together-with-others constitute humans' being. Such interdependence requires that each and everyone care to maintain and enhance life and society at large. This illustrates one of the major contradictions in human life, namely, that a life characterized by self-rule is also a life lived in interdependent relationships with others. This was a theme also discussed by Mead, "We are what we are through our relationship to others" (1934, p. 379), hence, consideration of others' interests and well-being is in one's own interest. Along the same line, Hume in his dispute with Kant's ethics based in rationality, argued that morality rests on the ability to reflective sentiment and on a balance between sympathy for the other and self-interest.

Similarly, the basic premise for the ethics of care developed by Noddings (1984) is that every human being is "existentially" dependent on others; one is both free and bound. Noddings traced the value of caring to our earliest memories of both caring and being cared for. These memories, the "longing for goodness" (p. 2); "our longing for caring—to be in that special relation— . . . provides the motivation for us to be moral" (p. 5); it constitutes the ethical ideal by which to live. Thus, caring is seen as a relation, which according to Noddings, is characterized by receptivity and reciprocity. The notion of receptivity is linked to the one-caring, "I see and feel with the other" (p. 30), which motivates one to be "at the service of the other" (p. 33). Reciprocity is linked to the one cared for, "being himself, this willing and unselfconscious revealing of self, is his major contribution to the relation" (p. 73). Thus, the reciprocal "gift" from the one cared for can be seen as the trust bestowed on the one caring. In Nodding's explication of an ethic of caring, caring appears as a relational value, "as a mark of a valuable kind of relation . . . [and] a characteristic way of being in the world" (Noddings, 1990, p. 28).

The concept of *transpersonal caring* developed by Watson (1988a) appears to be closely related to Noddings' concept of caring as a foundational and relational value. On the other hand, Watson also argues that caring is a moral ideal of nursing "whereby the end is protection, enhancement, and preservation of human dignity" (p. 29), however, she also discusses caring as a characteristic of the nurse; as an approach; and as a personal response, as nurse's acts or behavior on behalf of the patient.

WATSON'S THEORY OF HUMAN CARING

Jean Watson, with her book *Nursing: The Philosophy and Science of Caring* (1979), was one of the first nurse theorists to address the concept of caring as the focus of a nursing theory. In a recent article, Watson (1997) described this work as emerging from a "quest to bring new meaning and dignity to the world of nursing and patient care" (p. 49). The influence of biomedical sciences and the medical paradigm, she argued, limited the scope of care and was in dissonance with "nursing's paradigm . . . of caring-healing and health" (p. 49). The ten carative factors was the organizing framework of this first book and was developed further in her later work (Watson, 1988a; 1988b). The carative factors are seen as a combination of interventions and include: (a) The formation of a humanistic-altruistic system of values; (b) the instillation of faith-hope; (c) the cultivation of sensitivity to one's self and to others; (d) the development of a helping-trust relationship; (e) the promotion and acceptance of the expression of positive and negative feelings; (f) the systematic use of the scientific problem-solving method for decision making; (g) the promotion of interpersonal teaching-learning; (h) the provision for a supportive, protective, and (or) corrective mental, physical, sociocultural, and spiritual environment; (i) Assistance with gratification of human needs; and (j) the allowance for existential-phenomenological forces (1979, pp. 9–10).

According to Watson, these carative factors make up the *core of nursing*, which "refers to those aspects of nursing that are intrinsic to the actual nurse-patient/client process that produce therapeutic results in the person being served" (Watson, 1979, p. *xv*). Considering nursing as a therapeutic interpersonal process, as both scientific and artistic, Watson in her theory sought "to combine science with humanism" (p. *xvii*). The theoretical perspectives brought into the formulation and her explication of the carative factors were humanistic psychology, phenomenological philosophy, and existentialism (Watson, 1979; 1997). Furthermore, the value system on which these factors rest "was humanitarian, aesthetic, and spiritual" (Watson, 1997, p. 50). She argues that the carative factors provide "a structure and order for nursing phenomena" (p. 50), implicating that these are to be viewed as a nursing theory. Her concern is the human dimensions of nursing care, thus emphasizing the human-to-human relationship, characterized as a caring and healing relationship.

In *Nursing: Human Science and Human Care* (1988a), Watson posited her theory as reflecting an alternative world view of nursing that "will place nursing within a metaphysical context and establish nursing as a human-to-human care process with spiritual dimensions . . . " (p. 37), which is aimed at helping "persons gain higher degree of harmony within the mind, body, and soul [i.e., health] . . . " (p. 49). Accordingly, in this book, more emphasis is put on the moral, spiritual, and metaphysical dimensions of caring, for both patients and nurses. The caring relationship is seen as one that affects both the cared-for and the one caring, "in the caring transaction both are in a process of being and becoming" (p. 58), and "the nurse can enter into the experience of another person, and another can enter into the nurse's experience" (p. 60). In a recent publication Watson (1997) comments on the development this concept of transpersonal caring:

> [it] ultimately evokes and invites ontological development, a transformation of self . . . an integration of mind, body, and spirit . . . which is connected with all, elicits the spiritual and expanded views on what it means to be human: embodied spirit, both immanent and transcendent. . . . (p. 51)

It is clear that human beings, be it patients or nurses, now are viewed from a spiritual and metaphysical perspective. In accordance with this she comments on her work in this way " . . . it can be read as philosophy, ethic, or even paradigm or worldview" (p. 50). Thus, her carative factors, rather than providing a structure for nursing phenomena, as in 1979, are developed into a philosophical foundation from which nurses (and others) can develop a caring-healing relationship. However, because Watson only attributes these carative factors as the essential characteristics to be held and processed by the nurse in this so-called transpersonal caring, her position has not moved away from the notion of caring in nursing as a one-sided, normative approach. This position can be viewed as humanitarian but is not in full agreement with the major tenets of the generic notions of humanism.

Watson's theory is eclectic. She has pulled ideas from several sources in building her theoretical expositions. In addition to those already mentioned, major thoughts from pragmatism are evident, such as humans seen as experiencing subjects (subjective dimension) in ongoing change (interactive dimension) and the interconnectedness between humans and the world (interdependence dimension). Also, the influence of European philosophers, for example, Heidegger and Merleau-Ponty, is reflected in the use of concepts such as being-in-the world and the embodied spirit.

Thus, many of her positional statements reflect thoughts from pragmatism and humanism generally, however, her theory departs from mainstream humanism in the sense that major ideas from this philosophy are not reflected. The way this theory now is developed, rather than being seen as a humanistic nursing theory, it might be better named as an ontology of spirituality or spiritualism argued as a foundation for nursing practice. Since the Enlightenment era, humanism has opposed metaphysics and major strands of humanism are secular in their character. In humanism, rationality is seen as the definite characteristic of human beings, as a unique ability that furthers free will, decision making, and self-determination. The parts of nursing care that deal with how to preserve and facilitate patients' autonomy in decisions about their care are not reflected in the theory as it is now presented. Thus, the core value within humanism is over-shadowed by spiritualism in Watson's theory.

HUMANISM AND CARING IN NURSING—AN EXPOSITION

The philosophies of humanism and caring have been foundational to nursing throughout its history, shaping the basic character of nursing, namely, that nursing inherently is a moral practice. This practice is carried through in relation to persons in vulnerable and often dependent positions vis á vis the nurse. Thus, the nurse, being responsible for the patient's well-being while in the nurse's care, is implicitly a moral agent, and nursing practice is grounded in moral values. In this perspective three core values in humanism, human dignity, equality and freedom/autonomy will be discussed as to their conceptualization in nursing, as well as the concept of care. It will be argued that in nursing care must be seen as a moral motivation to act, with human dignity as a core value from which the values of autonomy and equality are derived.

The humanistic belief of the inherent worth of each person, his uniqueness, is a value held in high regard in nursing as reflected in the first injunction in The Code for Nurses, which states that the nurse unrestrictedly "provides services with respect for human dignity and the uniqueness of the client." Within humanism the fundamental status of persons, human dignity, is associated with the value of autonomy. This position within humanism can be traced to Kant, who argued "that respect for autonomy flows from the recognition that all persons have unconditional worth, each having the capacity to determine his or her own destiny" (Beauchamp & Childress, 1989, p. 71). Autonomy is considered as one of the most central values of a free society and is defined as "the condition of living according to laws one gives oneself, or negatively, not being under the control of another" (Haworth, 1986, p. 11). Kupfer (1990) argued that autonomy, conceived as a natural trait of human beings, as embodied in people, demands that every person is to be respected. This is an unearned respect in contrast to the respect one may be bestowed because one has done something extraordinarily well or something beneficial to others. Respecting a person implies to consider that person to have the same rights, privileges, or status as oneself. Hence, the value of equality is closely related to the value of autonomy. Furthermore, respecting a person requires that one helps that person to secure what is needed to realize these values in this person's situation in life. Also, "respect implies a realistic regard for the individual" (Kupfer, 1990, p. 51), which encompasses acceptance of and willingness to take the other's point of view with regard to the other's own interests, values, and purposes.

In humanism generally it is held that competence and rationality, the capacity for reasoning, is necessary to be considered a person, that is, having unique individual value (human dignity). Further, that rationality is a prerequisite for a person to be considered autonomous (Beauchamp & Childress, 1989). In the nursing context, such a position, that respect for persons is only linked to their rational capacity, is highly problematic. Often patients in nurses' care are in situations where their competence and reasoning capacity are limited either temporarily (unconscious patients) or permanently (senile dementia patients).

Therefore, the position taken here is that in nursing respect must be or rather is grounded in the inherent worth of individuals as human beings regardless of their capacities and characteristics (a nonsecular position). As stated by Kupfer (1990), a person is respected not "*because* of his individuality, we do respect him *in* his individuality. We take his interests, purposes, and degree of autonomy itself into account in the particular way we treat him" (p. 48). Because nurses respect the inherent worth of each patient, they uphold the value of equality through acting and interacting in regard to the degree of autonomy that is present. Looking at nursing practice one finds that nurses speak a normal language with demented patients; allow mentally ill patients to decide on issues within their capacity; interact with and give nursing care to the unconscious patient in the way they themselves would have wanted to be treated in a similar situation. As seen in nursing practice the value of the inherent worth of persons (human dignity) is not founded solely on the capacity to reason. Further, as the examples illustrate, in nursing autonomy and equality must be seen as rights that are derived from human dignity, rather than be regarded as foundational to human dignity, as within humanism.

The value of equality has two dimensions in nursing, one associated with the relationship between nurse and patient. Basic to nurses' acts and interactions with patients are the belief that patients and nurses have equal value as human beings, they are fellow human beings. In this the value of equality is an absolute right to be actualized in the nurse-patient relationship. The other dimension has to do with the relationship between patients in regard to their rights to equal share of privileges. The question of priorities has always been a part of nursing practice, however, in a time with cuts in economic resources to health care, ethical dilemmas related to actualizing the value equality are more pressing than ever. The value of equality cannot be seen as an absolute right in this regard, it is not possible to realize in the nursing service of today. Also the value of autonomy has two dimensions in nursing, one associated with the nurses' own autonomy, to exercise the right to decide on issues of patients' care that are in the nurses' domain, and to be heard as a competent partner in decisions on common ground for doctors and nurses. This is a right to be negotiated in a health care system in which physicians still dominate the power of decision making. The other dimension is the actualization of patients' rights to autonomy through collaboration and patients' active participation in decisions concerning themselves. However, in nursing autonomy cannot be seen as an absolute right of patients. In the interest of the good for some patients, the nurse may have to execute some form of paternalism, for example, forced suctioning of suicidal patients, overriding a patient's decision when this is harmful to him, and gentle prodding to make the patient change his mind in his best interest.

This issue brings in the value of altruism, which has been at the core of nursing throughout its history. However, lately it has re-emerged as the value of care. Care is a relatively new concept within contemporary moral philosophy and ethics (Blum, 1992). The reintroduction of care as a moral value came with Gilligan's (1982) research on women's reasoning and solutions to moral dilemmas, which identified a "moral voice" different from that of justice, the "voice of care." Historically, care was not used as a concept, nor seen as a value as such, but as a moral orientation, or rather as the foundation of morality, that which motivates to act morally. Among some philosophers, such as Schopenhauer, Hume, and Kierkegaard, altruism/compassion is regarded at the "cornerstone of ethics" (Blum, 1992). While compassion is considered as a sentiment underlying morality, altruism is generally defined as the regard for the well-being of others. Then a pertinent and significant question is: How does one know what is the good for the other?

In the nursing context, in which the good sought is the patient's health, well-being, or peaceful death, the nurse's professional knowledge and experience provide the basis from which to judge what is good for the actual patient. This is not sufficient, however, in nursing an understanding of what is "the good for the other" from the patient's perspective is also needed, either directly from the patient, relatives, or through reflective imagination, because without this understanding the desire for the patient's good may not be served. Hence, in nursing the moral foundation of altruism activates the realization of the values of equality and autonomy.

In the philosophy of caring explicated by Noddings, a reciprocal relationship between trust and caring is seen as foundational to human life. That is, the interdependence among individuals requires that everyone both care and trust to maintain and enhance life and society at large. One question surfaces, however: Are these explications of caring and trust in general human relationships a sufficient moral basis for nursing? One will argue that they are not. In contrast to caring and trust as ideals for conduct between people in general, in nursing these values have to be upheld and actualized by the nurse independent of patient participation and contribution to the relationship. Nurses are also responsible for nursing care to patients who lack the ability or have insufficient capacity to be actively involved in the relationship, for example, patients on ventilators, unconscious, or dying patients. That is, the conditional interdependence so basic to these values in general human relationships cannot always be upheld in the nursing context.

In conclusion, the philosophies of humanism and caring give a foundation for nursing as a moral practice, however, the basic values of these philosophies have to be reconceptualized to reflect and meet the realities of nursing practice as discussed above. Hence, care is best to be seen as a moral motivation to act in regard to the patients' well-being rather than as a relational value, that is, altruism is reintroduced in nursing. Also, in nursing respect for the patient as a person must be founded in the inherent worth of the individual regardless of capacity and competence, rather than in the notion of the rational autonomous individual. Furthermore, this value of human dignity is considered as the core value in nursing (Fagermoen, 1995; 1997). Hence, in nursing the values of equality and autonomy flow from the value of human dignity. Several studies of nurses have reported that nurses have patients' dignity in focus and purposely act through nursing care to preserve it when in jeopardy and to restore it when diminished. Then the value of human dignity in nursing can be considered as more than holding an attitude of respecting the individual's worth, as a value actualized in concrete acts to restore and maintain health and well-being of patients. Accordingly, the required physical care will, in certain situations, be primary to the relationship as such, and in emergency situations, for example, actions required to restore health and preserve dignity may conflict with other values, such as autonomy and reciprocal trust. Thus, in nursing these values are subsumed under the value of human dignity.

Finally, one moral imperative in humanism, to strive to understand the perspective of the other, is emphasized in professional nursing. To fulfill the aim of delivering care in the best interest of patients, professional nurses use a diverse base of knowledge. Together, professional knowledge; an understanding of what is good for the patient seen from the patient's perspective; previous experiences with other patients; intuition; and reflection on the specific patient's situation provide a basis for a general understanding of what it is like for patients. These sources of knowledge are constructing the foundation on which decisions are made in the patient's best interest, with the core value, human dignity, giving directions as to how the values of autonomy and equality are to be actualized in nursing care guided by an altruistic motivation.

The ontology embedded in the philosophy of humanism has been addressed as has its consequences for nursing practice. Also, epistemological issues have to be outlined in relation to the advancement of nursing knowledge. Accepting that humans are experiential, self-determining, and interpretative beings whose understanding of themselves, others, and situations is ongoing in interaction with the social and cultural context has definite implications in regard to how to investigate the human realm.

From the perspective of humanism, objective knowledge untangled by personal bias and personal perspective is not possible nor desirable to obtain, that is, the knowledge to be uncovered is relativistic in nature and the knowledge described is considered as approximations of truth. This position rests on two epistemological positions of pragmatism and hermeneutics. First, knowledge of a person's life is embedded in meanings individually constructed, that is, this knowledge is subjective and situated. Second, knowledge is also embedded in social and cultural values, artifacts, and practices; such knowledge is constructed as intersubjective meanings. Third, these views on human understanding and meanings also apply to the investigator and not only the person being investigated. Research in the human realm then requires a high degree of self-reflection on behalf of the investigator both in preparing and conducting a study to be attentive to foreknowledge, values, and attitudes that may color perceptions and interpretations. Further, multiple forms of inquiry are needed to uncover such knowledge whether it is the patients' or nurses' experiences and meanings or nursing practice as such. Phenomenological, ethnographic, grounded theory, and critical theory approaches employ methods of data collection, analysis, and interpretation that are in line with foundational ideas in humanism, however, each with different emphasis on which dimensions of understanding and meanings are focused on.

Humanism of the twentieth century, with a vision toward a new century, has to embrace not only the idea that humans must be allowed to exercise the power of self-determination but also at the same time the realization that in doing so there is a great danger to alienate and co-opt ourselves from the basic values of humanity. Thus, knowledge development in general and more specifically in such human practice disciplines as nursing, must be oriented to value identification and value determination as well as understanding and explanation. Nursing theories within the perspective of humanism then should begin with this paradoxical struggle in human nature.

REFERENCES

Abbagnano, N. (1972). Humanism. In J. Edwards (Ed.), *The encyclopedia of philosophy, Vol. 4* (pp. 69–72). New York: MacMillan.

Andic, M. (1991). What is Renaissance humanism? In D. Goicoechea, J. Luik, & T. Madigan (Eds.), *The question of humanism. Challenges and possibilities* (pp. 83–98). Buffalo, NY: Prometheus.

Baier, A. (1987). Hume, the women's moral theorist? In. E. F. Kittay & D. T. Meyers (Eds.), *Women and moral theory* (pp. 37–55). Totowa, NJ: Rowman & Littlefield.

Beauchamp, T., & Childress, J. (1989). *Principles of biomedical ethics* (3rd ed.). New York: Oxford University Press.

Blum, L. (1992). Altruism. In L. G. Becker & C. B. Becker (Eds.), *Encyclopedia of ethics: Vol. 1* (pp. 35–39). New York: Garland.

Bullock, A. (1985). *The humanist tradition in the West.* New York: Norton.

DeCarvalho, R. J. (1991). *The founders of humanistic psychology.* New York: Praeger.

Dewey, J. (1976/1916). Physical and social studies: Naturalism and humanism. In C. D. Sclosser (Ed.), *The person in education: A humanistic approach* (pp. 336–347). New York: MacMillan.

Diggins, J. P. (1994). *The promise of pragmatism: Modernism and the crisis of knowledge and authority.* Chicago: The University of Chicago Press.

Fagermoen, M. S. (1995). The meaning of nurses' work: A descriptive study of values fundamental to professional identity in nursing. (Doctoral dissertation,

University of Rhode Island, 1995). *Dissertation Abstracts International, 56/09-B*, 4814.

Fagermoen, M. S. (1997). Professional identity: Values embedded in meaningful nursing practice. *Journal of Advanced Nursing*, *25*, 434–441.

Fay, B., & Moon, J. D. (1994). What would an adequate philosophy of science look like. In: M. Martin & L. C. McIntyre (Eds.), *Readings in the philosophy of social science* (pp. 21–35). Cambridge, MA: The MIT Press.

Francis, R. P. (1991). The human person in American pragmatism. In D. Goicoechea, J. Luik, & T. Madigan (Eds.), *The question of humanism. Challenges and possibilities* (pp. 234–243). Buffalo, NY: Prometheus Books.

Gilligan, C. (1982). *In a different voice. Psychological theory and women's development.* Cambridge, MA: Harvard University Press.

Giorgi, A. (1970). *Psychology as a human science*. New York: Harper & Row.

Glaser, B., & Strauss, A. (1967). *The discovery of grounded theory*. Chicago: Aldine.

Goicoechea, D., Luik, J., & Madigan, T. (Eds.). (1991). *The question of humanism. Challenges and possibilities*. Buffalo, NY: Prometheus.

Haworth, L. (1986). *Autonomy: An essay in philosophical psychology and ethics*. New Haven, CT: Yale University Press.

Kolenda, K. (1995). Humanism. In R. Audi (Ed.), *The Cambridge dictionary of philosophy* (pp. 340–341). Cambridge, UK: Cambridge University Press.

Kupfer, J. H. (1990). *Autonomy and social interaction*. Albany, NY: State University of New York Press.

Kurtz, P. (1972). American philosophy. In J. Edwards (Ed.), *The encyclopedia of philosophy. Vol. 1* (pp. 83–93). New York: MacMillan.

Luik, J. (1991a). The question of humanism and the career of humanism. In D. Goicoechea, J. Luik, & T. Madigan (Eds.), *The question of humanism. Challenges and possibilities* (pp. 15–25). Buffalo, NY: Prometheus.

Luik, J. (1991b). An old question raised again: Is Kant an Enlightenment humanist? In D. Goicoechea, J. Luik, & T. Madigan (Eds.), *The question of humanism. Challenges and possibilities* (pp. 117–137). Buffalo, NY: Prometheus.

Madigan, T. (1991). Afterword: The answer to humanism. In D. Goicoechea, J. Luik, & T. Madigan (Eds.), *The question of humanism. Challenges and possibilities* (pp. 326–334). Buffalo, NY: Prometheus.

Maines, D. R. (1992). Pragmatism. In E. F. Borgatta & M. L.Borgatta (Eds.), *Encyclopedia of sociology* (pp. 1531–1536). New York: MacMillan.

Mead, G. H. (1934). *Mind, self, and society*. Chicago: The University of Chicago Press.

Mead, G. H. (1964a). Philantrophy from the point of view of ethics. In A. J. Reck (Ed.), *Selected writings: George Herbert Mead* (pp. 392–407). Chicago: University of Chicago Press.

Mead, G. H. (1964b). The definition of the physical. In A. J. Reck (Ed.), *Selected writings: George Herbert Mead* (pp. 25–59). Chicago: University of Chicago Press.

Morse, J. M., Bottorff, J. L., Neander, W. L., & Solberg, S. M. (1991). Comparative analysis of conceptualizations and theories of caring. *Image: Journal of Nursing Scholarship*, *23*, 119–126.

Morse, J. M., Solberg, S. M., Neander, W. L., Bottorff, J. L., & Johnson, J. L. (1990). Concepts of caring and caring as a concept. *Advances in Nursing Science*, *13*, 1–14.

Nerheim, H. (1995). *Vitenskap og kommunikasjon* (Science and communication). Oslo, Norway: Universitetsforlaget.

Nicolaisen, R. F. (1997). Eksistensialismen. In I. T. Tollefsen, H. Syse, & R. F. Nicolaisen (Eds.), *Tenkere og ideer* (pp. 524–537). (Existentialism. In: *Thinkers and ideas*.) Oslo, Norway: Ad Notam/Gyldendal.

Nightingale, F. (1859/1969). *Notes on nursing: What it is, and what it is not*. New York: D. Appleton.

Noddings, N. (1984). *Caring. A feminine approach to ethics & moral education*. Berkely, CA: University of California Press.

Noddings, N. (1990). Private caring and public care-giving: A proposal for synthesis. *Nytt om kvinneforskning*, *2*, 25–34.

Polkinghorne, D. (1983). *Methodology for the human sciences*. Albany, NY: State University of the New York Press.

Schwartz, M. A., & Wiggins, O. (1985). Science, humanism, and the nature of medical practice: A phenomenological view. *Perspectives in Biology and Medicine*, *28*, 331–361.

Skirbrekk, G., & Gilje, N. (1987). *Filosofi historie. Bind 2* (History of philosophy. Vol. 2). Oslo, Norway: Universitetsforlaget.

Thayer, H. S. (1972). *Pragmatism*. In J. Edwards (Ed.), *The encyclopedia of philosophy. Vol. 6* (pp. 430–436). New York: MacMillan.

Thompson, J. L. (1990). Hermeneutic inquiry. In L. Moody (Ed.), *Advancing nursing science through research. Vol. 2* (pp. 223–280). Newbury Park, CA: Sage.

Turner, J. H. (1986). *The structure of sociological theory* (4th ed.). Belmont, CA: Wadsworth.

Watson, J. (1979). *Nursing: The philosophy and science of caring*. Boston: Little, Brown.

Watson, J. (1988a). *Nursing: Human science and human care*. New York: National League for Nursing.

Watson, J. (1988b). New dimensions of human caring theory. *Nursing Science Quarterly, 1*, 175–181.

Watson, J. (1997). The theory of human caring: Retrospective and prospective. *Nursing Science Quarterly*, *10*, 49–52.

11

The Health/Illness Continuum*

Friedrich Balke

One of the major concerns in nursing science, as a field within the broader domain of health sciences, is conceptualizing health and illness. Conceptualization of health and illness is embedded in the broader context that determines the order of knowledge and the ways power is exercised in a society to deal with the matters of health and illness as social constructions. It is in this perspective that the notions of health, normality, illness, and pathologies as well as how societies develop processes to respond to such notions are examined in this chapter. The focus is in tracing and analyzing the genesis of radically different conceptualizations of health and illness in the modern era with the attendant emergence of power processes that become couched within the health-care processes (for example, hospitals) in modern times, and to examine how these are changing in the current scene.

NORMAL AND PATHOLOGICAL: THE INVENTION OF A NEW OPPOSITION TYPE

Ever since Immanuel Kant, philosophers have liked to pose the question of the condition of possible experience: they retreat, as it were, from what is empirically, that is, concretely perceived, thought, uttered and done, and ask what makes it possible for us to perceive, think, utter or do something in the way we do. This means that there is something present in people's everyday or lifetime actions of which those who carry out the actions are not conscious (just as it is not necessary to know any grammar rules to speak more or less grammatically correctly), but which

*Translated from German by Ellen Klein.

nevertheless functions in the background and serves as the base that supports a specific practice (practice is to be understood here in the widest sense).

In the following, I shall try, while taking a look at a phenomenon connected with these reflections which I shall call here provisionally "health sciences," to lay bare such a base: a base that begins to take form in the nineteenth century, supplants the classical conception of illness as an "accident," that is, a temporary or lethal defect, and creates a new image of the individual as someone who lives in illness: illness is always latently present in the individual (even when he is healthy), he is exposed to its risk (to the probability of falling ill) and must therefore subject himself to constant and essentially preventive self-observation and self-treatment. What are the changes in the order of knowledge and in the ways of exercising power that are responsible for health gradually ceasing to be the reference point of medicine (insofar as health is defined by the absence of illness and insofar as the body must decide, so to speak, between health and illness, insofar then as there is a real battle being waged between health or "nature" and illness for the body) and normality, or more precisely, the continuity from the normal and the pathological becoming its primary object? Or to put it another way, since we have not stopped distinguishing between healthy and ill: what is meant by this distinction when in the nineteenth century it is given an entirely new content, when it now acquires a sense originating from the horizon of the distinction between normal and pathological, which is of an entirely different nature? In the following, the "conditions for the change or interruption of meaning" will be described, that is, the conditions "under which the meaning fades [in our case: the old meaning of health and illness], thereby allowing something different to appear in its place" (Foucault, 1994a, p. 603), namely, the distinction between normal and pathological. In an interview dating from the year 1969, Michel Foucault explains the significance of this distinction for our culture with the following words:

> Every society establishes a series of opposition systems—between good and bad, permitted and forbidden, criminal and noncriminal, etc. All these oppositions, which are constitutive for every society, have been reduced in Europe today to the simple opposition of normal and pathological. This opposition is not only simpler than the others are, it also provides the advantage of allowing people to believe that there is a technique with which allows the pathological can be lead back to the normal. (Foucault, 1994a, p. 603)

In the following I shall try to answer the question of what makes this new opposition of normal and pathological so attractive, of what lends it its absorbing force. What are the qualities that allow an entire complex of traditional oppositions (good/bad, permitted/forbidden, criminal/non-criminal, etc.) with more or less moral, that is, qualitative, connotations to be translated into merely relative positional values on a graduated scale whose two poles (normality/abnormality) communicate with each other? What is the specific "simplicity" of this opposition in relation to the others spoken of by Foucault? Jürgen Link (1997a), who has presented the first comprehensive study of the archaeology of *normalism*, provides the following provisional answer, which will have to be developed further on: The simplicity of this new distinction lies in its one-dimensionality. No matter how heterogeneous, discontinuous or multidimensional a particular range of phenomena is and regardless of its qualitative characteristics, the normalizing strategy consists in ascribing to this multifissured territory a parallel level that allows all possible positions, even the most extreme and improbable, to be thought of as homogeneous and continuous. The establishment of such *normal fields* is at the same time the prerequisite for increasing the performance of normalizing interventions, which are to a large extent abstracted from the qualitative peculiarities of their intervention space so as to increase their ability to be technically manipulated.

In a first step the question to be addressed is: What changes in the order of knowledge made possible this modern normalist perspective, which in the nineteenth century began its triumphant advance through the entire realm of human scientific knowledge? Following this epistemological inquiry, which will lead us into the middle of the field of treating and dealing with patients, the way this very new knowledge type interacts with equally new *power processes* will be analyzed. These processes will not only be viewed under the aspect of how normalist knowledge and normalist techniques are applied, but also in particular under the aspect of how such knowledge and techniques are generated, that is, their discursive productivity.

Let us begin with the first question, which requires a brief excursion to the biomedical knowledge complex that was forming in the nineteenth century. The distinction between normal and pathological conceived in the field of physiopathology undergoes as early as the beginning of the nineteenth century a critical transformation, at the end of which a qualitative difference is replaced by a quantitative difference. Foucault alludes to this process when he emphasizes the "simplicity" of this new opposition, and we shall see that the increasing use of technology involved with it is also connected with this quality. The French science historian George Canguilhem showed in his study *On the Normal and the Pathological* published originally in 1943 how in the medical science of that age classical ontological pathology was replaced by a theory that emphasized the continuity and homogeneity in the sick and healthy states. While ontological theory envisions "in disease, or better, in the experience of being sick [. . .] a polemical situation: either a battle between the organism and a foreign substance, or an internal struggle between opposing forces" (Canguilhem, 1978, p. 12), the new conception of illness reduces illness to a mere deviation from health, a measurable change in intensity of the "normal" state. The ill state was conceived by the French doctor Broussais in his treatise *De l'irritation et de la folie,* appearing in 1827 and based on the model of (mental) *irritation*, which according to Broussais is nothing other than "a normal stimulation in an exaggerated form." The phenomena that are the object of pathological examination are not different in nature, but only in degree from those of physiology. This nosology[1] of continuity, developed further with certain modifications and radicalized by Claude Bernard, was taken up by Auguste Comte, the founding father of sociology, who generalized Broussais's principle to an axiom also applicable to social processes.

> "Our famous fellow citizen, Broussais," should be thanked, said Comte in his fortieth lecture of the "Cours de Philosophie Positive," for his courageously advocated view that the pathological state is not at all radically different from the physiological state, with regard to which—no matter how one looks at it—it can only constitute a simple extension going more or less beyond the higher or lower limits of variation proper to each phenomenon of the normal organism, without ever being able to produce really new phenomena. (Canguilhem, 1978, p. 19)

Even philosophers of Nietzsche's caliber were fascinated by the possibilities of knowledge that the qualitative leveling of the former antagonism between health and illness, and the reduction of pathology to the status of a complementary discipline of physiology seemed to afford. Thus we read in an entry from his posthumous works of the 1880s, which is followed by a longer key quotation from Claude Bernard's *Leçon sur la chaleur animale* translated by Nietzsche: "It is the value of all morbid states that they show us under a magnifying glass certain states that are normal—but not easily visible when normal" (as cited in Canguilhem, 1978, p. 15). The Bernard quotation translated by Nietzsche reads:

> Health and sickness are not essentially different, as the ancient physicians and some practitioners even today suppose. One must not make of them

> distinct principles or entities that fight over the living organism and turn it into their arena. That is silly nonsense and chatter that is no good any longer. In fact, there are only differences in degree between these two kinds of existence: the exaggeration, the disproportion, the nonharmony of the normal phenomena constitute the pathological state. (as cited in Nietzsche, 1968, p. 29)

The morbid condition is revealed to modern doctors then as a deviation in a chain of continuity ("differences in degree") from the individual's healthy existence. Modern medicine functions by means of a differential method, a method that differentiates degrees—it is not by chance that "differential diagnosis" has become its most important instrument. The term *normal* is now defined with reference to statistically obtained averages and describes a range of acceptable deviation (obtained by setting limits and tolerance thresholds); *pathological* means in the region on the other side of the normality line, which itself is always dynamic and only temporary, that is, shiftable within a continuum. In any case, no insurmountable wall exists between the two conditions, but only a variable threshold. The process of making a fundamental discontinuity into a continuity consists in constructing a common axis of comparability between two conditions (health/illness) hitherto viewed as qualitatively different. After a period of time in which the field of pathologies had been comprehended with the aid of a taxonomic model that distinguished between perfect realizations of a type and corrupt or "monstrous" forms, the doctor's gaze was completely reorganized at the beginning of the nineteenth century:

1. First, it was no longer the gaze of any observer, but that of a doctor supported and justified by an institution, that of a doctor endowed with the power of decision and intervention.
2. The gaze was no longer "bound by the narrow grid of structure (form, arrangement, number, size), but could and should grasp colors, variations, tiny anomalies, always receptive to the deviant" (medicine of deviations instead of medicine of types).
3. It was no longer satisfied with ascertaining what was directly visible or self-evident, but inferred "chances and risks": a calculating, prognosticating gaze (Foucault, 1973, p. 89).

Canguilhem has called attention to the significant etymological circumstance that the term "normal" could be attested as early as 1759, whereas "normalized" was encountered for the first time only in 1834—a time when the debate on the new, positive pathology was at its first peak (Canguilhem, 1978, p. 151). We have now reached the point where it becomes clear that there is more to the question with the new distinction of normal/pathological than only acceptance of a changed medical procedure of discovery and treatment. At stake is nothing less than the question of power itself. In order to be able to comprehend our contemporary societies it is necessary that we divorce ourselves from some of our habits of thought regarding power that we have become accustomed to. Most important is that we abandon the notion of power as something that functions essentially negatively or repressively. According to this conception, the power that is generally localized in the state is essentially concerned with preventing, repressing, skimming off profit, suppressing. It manifests itself in the legal system or in laws whose function consists in formulating prohibitions and threatening sanctions when these rules and regulations are violated. This classic power type, as it was characteristic of the early modern "sovereignty societies" and thus of the founding and establishment phase of the modern territorial states that were equipped with central power, culminates in the right over life and death of its subjects. The symbol of sovereign power is the sword.

However, long before the French Revolution, which sweeps away the social foundation of absolutistic power, entirely new power mechanisms develop in European societies. Their peculiarity lies in the fact that they are no longer played out at the level of the law—or when this level is entered upon, the way the law functions is fundamentally changed. We actually live in a society in which the power of the law is not simply diminishing, but the law is being integrated into the mechanism of completely differently functioning power processes: Foucault classifies these new power processes under the heading of *norm* (as opposed to *law*). Symptomatic for this transformation are the difficulties which arise within the heart of justice (criminal justice) itself when the task for which it was created has to be carried out, namely passing judgement, pronouncing a sentence, and determining the punishment for the delinquent. Punishments, of course, continue to be carried out, but in actual practice the function and meaning of punishment have fundamentally changed. This can be recognized by the fact that the status of criminals is being brought closer and closer to that of the ill, or more specifically, to that of the mentally ill, and the sentence for crime is understood as a *therapeutic* prescription.

As the process of arriving at a sentence for crime conforms more and more to medical-psychiatric diagnostics (or these diagnostic procedures attain greater importance in criminal proceedings, noticeably weaken the sharp opposition of guilty/not guilty, and allow all kinds of reduced culpability to arise), the ritual of punishing also acquires a new meaning, namely a therapeutic one: "We punish, but this is a way of saying that we wish to obtain a cure. Today, criminal justice functions and justifies itself only by this perpetual reference to something other than itself, by this unceasing reinscription in non-juridical [in fact *normalizing*, F.B.] systems" (Foucault, 1979, p. 22). From the moment that we are dealing with a *normalizing society* that interprets the entirety of its moral and legal codes in light of the distinction between normal and pathological, medicine becomes the prime discipline, precisely because it is the science of the normal and the pathological.

As the new power processes become detached from the law, they do not by any means fall back to the level of "brute" force; to understand them, rather, it is necessary to use language that comprehends them as *forces*. What does it mean then when the central activity of the modern powers is characterized by the term normalization? As opposed to normality, which is perceived as a fixed condition that is legally defined and guaranteed by police force, normalization as a category of process accentuates first of all the character of power as a relation between forces: a force does not come into contact with an object or a thing and destroy or change its form, but with another force that it cannot control without making itself dependent on the potency, the inner capacity of that force. Power relinquishes to a certain extent its vertical privilege, it is no longer situated over or in front of its field of activity, but taps into the forces it is trying to command, or more precisely, control. When we say that the new power is a relation between forces, then this simultaneously excludes the notion that it materializes in a sovereign form (for instance, the state). It no longer occurs in the singular (power does not form an opposition to powerlessness), it ceases to be a privilege of the powerful so that the question of who possesses it becomes meaningless. Power is not *possessed*, it is *exercised*; it does not exist in and of itself, it is operative. To stimulate, prompt, produce are the categories of the new power which "has taken possession of the lives of individuals, of individuals as living bodies," and both as individual bodies and as generic bodies. "A power bent on generating forces, making them grow, and ordering them, rather than one dedicated to impending them, making them submit, or destroying" (Foucault, 1981, p. 136). It does this by developing an entire series of disciplines for the individual body which serve to "increase its capabilities," "exploit its strengths" and integrate it into effective and economical control systems; furthermore, by subjecting the body of the population to various interventions which are supposed to regulate all aspects of collective life: reproduction, birth and death rates, health standards, life expectancy, migration, settlement, and so forth. Included within such disciplines would be nursing.

What Michel Foucault calls the "bio-power" has two sides or two focal points: any *body* and any *population*—the individual physical performance and the collective life processes. A power such as this, which is supposed to guarantee and enhance life, "needs continuous regulatory and corrective mechanisms. It is no longer a matter of bringing death into play in the field of sovereignty, but of distributing the living in the domain of value and utility. Such a power has to qualify, measure, appraise, and hierarchize, rather than display itself in its murderous splendor; it does not have to draw the line that separates the enemies of the sovereign from his obedient subjects; it effects distributions around the norm" (Foucault, 1981, p. 144), a formulation which makes the norm clearly recognizable as an average value that is derived from a comparative field and statistically obtained.

In his systematic analytics of disciplinary power, that power which selects the individual body as its target, Foucault, following the treatise literature on the subject which he makes use of, now returns to the "repressive" conceptualization of subduing, teaching, training, etc., although on the other hand it is exactly this disapproval of the "repression hypothesis" that is one of his main concerns. And so he says of "disciplinary power," to which the body is exposed:

> It does not link forces together in order to reduce them; it seeks to bind them together in such a way as to multiply and use them. Instead of bending all its subjects into a single uniform mass, it separates, analyses, differentiates, and carries its procedures of decomposition to the point of necessary and sufficient single units. [. . .] Discipline 'makes' (*'fabrique'*) individuals. (Foucault, 1979, p. 170)

The disciplinary power described by Foucault has an *individualizing* effect—and starting with this quality is the best way to approach the concept of normality. For a power can only have an individualizing effect if it assumes a different relationship to deviations from a given norm, if it responds to these deviations not by excluding or perhaps even destroying the deviator, but by employing a complex technique that allows the deviation to be regulated and that possibly even uses it to intensify bodily functions ("immunology") or the function of an institutional connection involving the bodies. To normalize means above all: not to eliminate, but to observe minutely, to differentiate and to recombine. The new power is attracted to deviations and contributes actively, as shown by the example of the evolution of modern sexuality analyzed by Foucault, to their growth and proliferation. The disciplinary power has an intensifying effect on deviation.

THE BIRTH OF THE HOSPITAL—FOUCAULTIAN CRITIQUE

Foucault analyzed how discipline functions in a series of typical organizations of modern societies: in addition to the army and factory, also in the school, the prison, psychiatry and the hospital. In the second part of my reflections I would like to take up the particularly interesting case of the hospital and show that the meeting of medicine and hospital, however it is to be judged, is an event whose occurrence is due solely to the new power mechanisms—that a political (and not a medical!) technology forms the basis of what we have known ever since as the hospital. One has the impression nowadays that hospitals are losing their privileged status as a place for treating the ill, a process that, as I expect, many who are involved in patient treatment and care observe with mixed feelings and perhaps even support actively. There is without a doubt a crisis of the hospital because there is also a crisis of the other milieus of confinement in whose framework modern power functions. And is not the academic establishment of nursing studies a response to the erosion of the hospital model, and does this not reflect the entire ambivalence of such processes of crisis insofar as some people primarily expect that by turning nursing into a scientific discipline there will be a revitalization of the hospital in the form of economization or increased efficiency (without touching its underlying power type), while others seek to supplement or perhaps even replace it with other forms of patient treatment and care?

A look at the phase of formation of the classic hospital model teaches us that it is not primarily new medical knowledge or knowledge of nursing that will accelerate the transformation of this model, but rather the attempt to use and intensify the crisis of the normalizing power already in process to seek solutions that have neither the character of a big, illusory "revolution" nor that of a reformation in which the goal of stabilizing the old model is pursued by enabling a series of controlled changes (cf. Foucault, 1994b, p. 547). The apologists of the status quo have in common with the revolutionary nostalgists that they always make the question of goals the focus of their politics—defining goals is the real strength of the experts of goal reflection, that is, of the intellectuals of the classic type. However, the history of the hospital in particular shows what cannot be made clear enough: No one wanted it, but nevertheless its triumphant progress has been uncheckable. The notion that sociocultural evolution, that is, the emergence and general acceptance of something new in the social world, results from the actions of strongly motivated and unerring individuals has had to be dismissed in the meantime (Luhmann, 1997, p. 456). Mutations occur through the exploitation of happy coincidences—and this means: They are just as fortuitous as the events by which they are occasioned. Coincidence is not concerned with goals and purposes. The question: "What do you really want?" is therefore invariably the question posed by reasonable people, legislators, technocrats, and governments, and addressed to those who want to play a different game (Foucault, 1994b, p. 544). History is not an object of the will, but of the coincidence of different factors or forces which none of the participants control. The task of the genealogist, as defined by Nietzsche, is not to go back to the pure origin of things before time, but to their emergence (*Entstehungsherd*). The beginning is neither true nor good nor beautiful, so it is neither reasonable nor at all simple, but differential, many-faceted and in a higher sense amoral.

Even those who benefited most from the establishment of the hospital, the doctors, only made it their goal after conditions for making it possible were already given by the coming about of a favorable situation unique in history, a meeting of various "coincidences." In any case, it can be said that the hospital is not an invention of doctors. It can be concluded from this that whatever will come after the hospital or shake the central role this institution plays in the process of medical treatment, and this will not take place without a fundamental change in the established scheme of the division of labor and in the way the participants in the medical process (doctors, nursing staff, patients) comprehend their roles, will not be the work of those who have been underprivileged so far in this process. How did the process of the medicalization of the hospital come about and what developments at the present time justify our suspicion that a loss of the medical privileges claimed by the hospital for itself is not far off, a loss extremely double-edged in its significance because it can lead to a universalization of the hospital model beyond the walls of the hospital as well as to a turning away from the power mechanisms and their structuring effect on the professions (dominance of medicine over nursing) that made the hospital model possible in the first place.

When I speak of the medicalization of the hospital, then this means that throughout its history the hospital was not always a place where a specifically medical influence was exerted on the patients. Until far into the eighteenth century there was in Europe indeed no area of contact between the practice of doctors and the hospital. Around 1760, the idea of using the hospital as an instrument for healing patients came into existence for the first time. In the Middle Ages and in early modern times the hospital did not function as a therapeutic instrument. The hospitals had the function of collecting the sick (and not only the sick) and preventing their coming into contact with their surroundings in order to hinder dangerous processes of infection (of physical as well as of "moral" nature). For the most part, the hospital was even more of a relief institution for the poor than for the sick (and for the sick only insofar as they were poor at the same time). The relief was of both material and spiritual nature. As a rule, it occurred only when a poor person was dying and consisted entirely in providing physical, but above all spiritual relief during the dying process. It was not by chance that the personnel of the hospitals was made up predominantly of members of orders who hoped to promote the salvation of the "patient's" soul as well as that of their own by their activities.

Conversely, at this time medicine is not a hospital medicine and not a hospital profession. The medicine of the Middle Ages takes place outside of the hospitals and is therefore a deeply individualistic practice consisting of three elements: the doctor, the illness, and the "nature." The doctor's intervention in the illness centered around the idea of the *crisis*. The crisis was that moment in which in the sick person's healthy nature and the evil afflicting him stood face to face in battle against each other. In this fight between the (good) nature and the illness it was the doctor's task to observe the signs, predict the development of the fight, and to do everything within his power to bring about the triumph of health and nature over the illness. Let us recall the words of Claude Bernard translated by Nietzsche precisely regarding that dualistic ontology which makes illness and health into two distinct principles or entities that are involved in an unrelenting struggle, in a real battle from which only one of the two sides can emerge as the victor. "That is nonsense and foolish talk and not good for anything," (as cited in Nietzsche, 1968, p. 29), wrote Bernard without giving an account, however, of the causes leading to the loss of evidence for this polemic schema of medical practice. The treatment, which takes the form of a battle, is invariably reduced to the individual relationship between the doctor and the patient. The idea of making extensive observations in the heart of the hospital to obtain a systematic basis of comparison and thus arrive at a differential ascertainment of the illness was not an element of medical practice for a very long time.

This only changes at the moment as the hospital becomes a political-economic annoyance in the eyes of the representatives of the public order. There is a mixture of all kinds of outcasts collected in it. It is true that they are all poor, but not all in the same way: beggars, mad people, sick people, prostitutes, and criminals constitute a highly diffuse social ensemble whose control is seen as a growing problem by the political authorities. The first hospital reform, occurring in France in the final years of the seventeenth century, was not of civil, but of military hospitals and of hospitals located in the port cities, which above all were places of economic disorder. They were important trading centers for goods smuggled into the country by sailors who feigned illness in order to slip by the customs officials. It was especially the military hospitals, however, that required a new, and specifically medical regimen to reduce the high mortality rate of soldiers outside of battle, after the costs for their education and upkeep had become a financial policy issue of the highest order following the introduction of firearms. The reorganization of the military hospitals was not based on a new medical technique, but on a technique that was essentially political, for which Foucault reserved the term disciplines. I have already pointed out the essentially productive character of this new power process and its simultaneously differentiating (dissolving impenetrable, complex conglomerates) and homogenizing (creating a new, "analytical space") effects, so it only remains for me to specify the most important registers of disciplinary power, while taking into consideration the invention of the hospital as a medical-therapeutic instrument in the following three accounts:

1. Discipline is first of all the art of spatial distribution of individuals: "Each individual has its own place; and each place its individual. Avoid distributions in groups; break up collective dispositions; analyse confused, massive or transient pluralities" (Foucault, 1979, p. 143). Medical surveillance of illness and infection goes hand in hand with other controls—first and foremost, the management of things (even before curing patients): registration of medications used, ascertainment of the actual number of patients, regulation of their comings and goings, creation of special categories for certain patients, continuous recording of medical histories, etc. (Foucault, 1979, p. 144). In summary: "The first of the great operations of discipline is, therefore, the constitution of '*tableaux vivants*', which transform the confused, useless or dangerous multitudes into ordered multiplicities. The drawing up of 'tables' was one of the great

problems of the scientific, political and economic technology of the eighteenth century" (Foucault, 1979, p. 148).

2. Installing discipline requires the establishment of the *coercive gaze*: In the course of the classical period "observatories of human multiplicity" (Foucault, 1979, p. 171) come into being. These are realized architecturally so that they enable a vantage point from which one can see without being seen (the ideal of the panoptic view). It is not sufficient merely to observe the patients from time to time, but rather they must be under permanent surveillance because it is only in this way that they can be exposed to knowledge that will change them. The most important instrument of this permanent surveillance of patients therefore becomes the ritual of the visit. Rather than a ritual, it would be more appropriate to speak of an *examination* that establishes over patients a visibility "through which one differentiates them and judges them" (Foucault, 1979, p. 184). As Foucault writes,

> [In this] slender technique are to be found a whole domain of knowledge, a whole type of power. The decisive factor for the epistemological 'thaw' of medicine at the end of the eighteenth century was the organization of the hospital as an 'examining' apparatus.[2] The ritual of the visit was its most obvious form. [. . .] The old form of inspection [which, moreover, was conducted by a physician from outside, who otherwise had no part in the leadership of the hospital, F.B.], irregular and rapid, was transformed into a regular observation that placed the patient in a situation of almost perpetual examination. This had two consequences: in the internal hierarchy, the physician, hitherto an external element, begins to gain over the religious staff and to relegate them to a clearly specified, but subordinate role in the technique of the examination; the category of the 'nurse' then appears; while the hospital itself, which was once little more than a poorhouse, was to become a place of training and of the correlation of knowledge; it represented a reversal therefore of the power relations and the constitution of a corpus of knowledge. The 'well-disciplined' hospital became the physical counterpart of the medical 'discipline'; this discipline could now abandon its textual character and take its references not so much from the tradition of author-authorities as from a domain of objects perpetually offered for examination. (Foucault, 1979, p. 185)

If it is possible to determine accurately the historical moment when specific nursing functions which play a "clearly specified, but subordinate role in the technique of the examination" in the hospital emerge, then the fact that the nursing staff as well as the "dominating" physician enter by virtue of their roles into complicity with disciplinary power can be recognized; at the same time however, the potential fracture point of the medical-nursing, or in a word, of the therapeutic solidarity is also recognizable, a fracture point that becomes virulent at the moment the consensus regarding the power-knowledge nexus, which makes possible and guarantees the hospital, crumbles and the nursing staff become aware that what they do must become the object of a specific knowledge that does not play a merely supplementary role in the techniques of producing medical knowledge.

3. Disciplinary power demands a permanent register, it is essentially a "power of writing" (Foucault, 1979, p. 189) and inspires entirely new recording and documentation methods whose function consists in enabling comparative fields to be organized—

> . . . making it possible to classify, to form categories, to determine averages, to fix norms: The hospitals of the eighteenth century, in particular, were great laboratories for scriptuary and documentary methods. The keeping of registers, their specification, the modes of transcription from one to the other, their circulation during visits, their comparison during regular meetings of doctors and administrators, the transmission of their data to centralizing bodies (either at the hospital or at the central office of the poorhouse), the accountancy of diseases, cures, deaths, at the level of a hospital, a town and even of the nation as a whole formed an integral part of the process by which hospitals were subjected to the disciplinary régime. (Foucault, 1979, p. 190)

Through maximum individualization of the individual to a "case," a comparative system was created, "that made possible the measurement of overall phenomena, the description of groups, the characterization of collective facts, the calculation of the gaps between individuals, their distribution in a given 'population' " (Foucault 1979, p. 190). Individualization in the normalist sense is a quasi-police function that consists in ascertaining small and even smaller differences between individuals, thereby constituting them to objects of knowledge that can be further and further broken down into components. In the context of disciplinary power, individualization means as much as unrestrained mass production of data. The hospital that is disciplined this way is the most important pivot between disciplinary power aiming at the individual body and the global regulation of the collective body (the population) undertaken by bio-power. The hospital attains such outstanding significance for the development of the human sciences because for the first time the "small techniques of notation, of registration, of constituting files, of arranging facts in columns and tables that are so familiar to us now," which were tested in its space, have transformed the individual (and not just the species) in his irreducible uniqueness into an object of knowledge and of a science that could be rightfully called "clinical science": "the problem of the entry of individual description, of the cross-examination, of anamnesis, of the 'file' into the general functioning of scientific discourse" (Foucault, 1979, p. 191).

Disciplinary power functions in an individualizing way and thus reinforces deviations in two ways:

- First of all, in contrast with traditional power it is concerned with ordinary individuality, which for a long time "remained below the threshold of description." In the age of disciplinary power, the chronicle becomes fundamental and loses its classic heroizing function: "It is no longer a monument for future memory, but a document for possible use" (Foucault, 1979, p. 191).
- Secondly, it is an active individualizing power that makes the *individual difference* which it is interested in perceptible in the first place or else produces it. The individual difference is not already present before the intervention of the power and only in need of representation, it is rather that disciplinary power creates the individual difference—namely to the extent in which it is successful in giving it a means of articulation.

FROM CONTROL TO SELF CONTROL

There are many indications that we are in a period of transition from one power regime to another. It is not by chance that Foucault's analytics of disciplinary power concentrate on the nineteenth century, the period when this power type receives its classic stamp. "but it is obvious that in the future we will have to divorce ourselves from the disciplinary society of today" (Foucault, 1994b, p. 533). It appears that we are now in the middle of this future in which the crisis of disciplinary society is taking place. However, the transformation which we are witnessing must not be imagined as happening according to the convenient pattern of a surgical incision. The strengths of the inventions of disciplinary power were demonstrated above all in the way these inventions became connected with a series of already existing important social institutions, to which they gave a completely new meaning, as we could observe in the example of the transformation from the classical to the modern hospital. The disciplinary power does not possess an essence of its own, it is thoroughly operative and therefore cannot be equated with one of the institutions which it uses as its milieu of realization. And what if the future of the disciplinary society, that is to say our future, consists in the disciplines, the procedures for producing the individual difference, becoming increasingly deinstitutionalized when they take their milieus "piggy-back," so to speak, in order to be even more variable and adaptable than they could ever be within the framework of the classic fundamental institutions (army, factory, school, clinic, prison)? To what forces is the fully evolved disciplinary power exposed in our time?

To answer this question, or more modestly put, to contribute elements to its answer, it should be remembered that Foucault links his analytics of the disciplines to the problem of space in a fundamental way: The disciplines replace the impenetrable "mixed spaces" (remember the function of the "old" hospital as a collecting basin of poverty) with living tableaus, "which transform the confused, useless or dangerous multitudes into ordered multiplicities" (Foucault, 1979, p. 148). The creation of a serial space is the prerequisite for the individualizing effect of normalizing power: every element in its place, no roving around or vagabonding. The main thing is to measure distances, to determine levels, to record exceptional features and harmonize the differences with each other beneficially. In the age of disciplinary power, the individualizing effect of normality can only be achieved within a closed space, a "milieu of confinement," which lends it its specifically repressive character. The dissolving or individualizing effects of the disciplines develop systematically within the already existing milieus of confinement, in which "abnormalities" are concentrated.

While it was characteristic for predisciplinary power—as can be seen from the exclusion rituals with which leprosy was responded to—that it invariably worked with a massive and dichotomizing boundary drawn between the one and the other, that it excluded spatially or simply eliminated by force what was deviant instead of comprehending it as an object of potential knowledge and therapeutic intervention (the sword as the symbol of power in the "sovereignty societies"), the disciplines respond to disorder by including the "source of trouble" into the order, or more precisely: They respond with a strategy of forming enclaves rather than exclaves. The "dangerous mixtures" are confined (rather than forcefully expelled)—albeit at the price of subjecting them to a more intense and, as it were, more branched power, a power that replaces the friend/enemy distinction, the "massive and binary distinction between one set of people and another" with different kinds of separations and individualizing distributions: differentiation instead of exile-enclosure (Foucault, 1979, p. 198). However, the decomposition of evil does not come about without exclusion, which now takes place within society and is localized institutionally and not least architecturally. It is as if the new power did not trust itself for a minute and therefore adopts the familiar milieus of confinement from the old power.

However, it is precisely these milieus of confinement that are at stake in modern times. The power of the norm(alization) is becoming radical to the same extent that it is gaining faith in itself and getting along without the walls of the milieus it has functioned within up to this time. For the future of the deinstitutionalized disciplines, Gilles Deleuze, the French philosopher and friend of Michel Foucault, has suggested the term *control societies*. Controls are virtually disciplines in the state of vagabondage. We must remember in connection with this term that Foucault had already pointed out *control*—the examining of behavior with a microscope—as an essential characteristic of the monitoring power that operates within the milieus of confinement. What is happening now is that this element is virtually being set free and its function changed: Control is separating from the architecture of the hierarchy to which it is still tied in the age of disciplinary power, it is ceasing to be a vertical privilege. Despite all preferences for circular architectures, disciplinary power was not able to manage without the model of the pyramid, the centralization at the top (Foucault, 1979, p. 174). Control in the age of control societies is being subjected on the other hand to a decentering and deterritorializing movement that can no longer be restricted to the space of a "total institution" (Goffman, 1963). Even before Goffman it was thought to be true that surveillance does not come only from above, but also from below and from the side: a network that pervades the institution, as Foucault wrote, with the effects of power: "supervisors, perpetually supervised" (Foucault, 1979, p. 177).

> We are in the process of entering 'control' societies that, strictly speaking, are no longer disciplinary societies. It is not seldom that Foucault is regarded as a philosopher of disciplinary societies and their fundamental technique, confinement (not only hospital and prison, but also school, factory, barracks). In reality, though, he is among the first who say that we are in the process of departing from disciplinary societies, that they are no longer

> our reality. We are entering control societies that no longer function by internment but rather by constant control and direct communication. [. . .] Certainly, there is constant talk of the prison, school, and hospital: these institutions are in a state of crisis. They are indeed in a state of crisis, but this is precisely because they are anachronistic. New types of sanctioning, education and nursing are gradually developing. Open hospitals, home nursing etc. are no longer new. And it is foreseeable that education will not remain a closed milieu that distinguishes itself from the closed milieu of the working world, but that both will disappear and a terrible kind of permanent further education will appear in their place, a continuous control to which the worker—secondary school pupil or the executive—university student will be subjected. [. . .] In a control regime you are never finished with anything. (Deleuze, 1990a, p. 236f)

The control societies, whose dawn we are now experiencing, are freeing the disciplines from the corset of the milieus of confinement and enabling them to penetrate all of society. This expansion of their area of activity requires, however, a change in their mode of action. Deleuze expressed the difference in how controls are exerted using the following image: "The confinements are different kinds of molds, casting molds, whereas the controls are a modulation, they are like a self-forming mold that changes from one moment to the next or a sieve whose meshes vary from one point to another" (Deleuze, 1990b, p. 242). Foucault, we remember, had said of disciplinary power that it has a normalizing effect, that it does not simply separate what is permitted from what is forbidden, but ascertains the individual's respective position differentially in a system of degrees of normality (and what is more: ascertains it again and again) (Foucault, 1979, p. 184), and judges it according to its distance from the norm, which is a statistically obtained and temporary average value.

In his *Essay on Normalism* (*Versuch über den Normalismus*), Jürgen Link (1997) deals with the possible reasons for Foucault's unresolved ambivalence with regard to his own use of the theoretical term. Normalism, as it in the nineteenth century comes to comprehend central sectors of modern society, is not a uniform phenomenon; it appears in the form of two rivaling strategies that try to form fields of normality in different ways, but become effective always jointly. Normalism is namely itself a part of the problem that it is supposed to solve: If Broussais's principle of the fundamental continuity between normal and abnormal phenomena is really valid, the fear that basically anyone can cross the boundary, which is no longer ontologically established, that is, no longer perceptible for everyone to the same extent, must become virulent. The *protonormalists*, as Links calls them, react to this typically modern anxiety of an irreversible denormalization by employing the strategy of maximum compression of the zone of normality and a correspondingly strict semantic and symbolic marking of the boundaries of normality; the *flexible-normalist* strategy on the other hand, which becomes extremely prevalent in western societies after the Second World War ("permissive society"), strives for a maximum expansion and dynamic quality of the zone of normality, for which purpose it always fixes a temporary boundary of normality, that is, keeps it reversible and, figuratively speaking, does not constitute it as a wall, but as a transitional space or passage. This tug-of-war situation between the two strategies is taken into account by Foucault—without his conceptualizing it—insofar as his description of the new power order constantly oscillates between dynamic-open and repressive categories (disciplines, training, etc.).

The Janus-facedness of the normalizing societies is founded upon the paradoxical status of the boundary: Namely, if normalism is characterized on the one hand by the fact that its boundaries are invariably precarious and provisional because it presupposes a fundamental continuity between normal and abnormal phenomena and does not tolerate any qualitative (that is, anything not fundamentally within reach of the normalizing influence) differences or antagonisms, then it cannot on the other hand be separated from a boundary politics because the activity of normalism has precisely the purpose of providing protection against the risk of irreversible denormalization (that is, of absolute abnormalities), a risk associated with the normal reproduction modus of modern societies. Although normalism has thus lost all respect for inviolable, qualitative boundaries (which possess to a certain degree the status of tabus), since it recognizes only flexible limits in a continuum, it is still thoroughly convinced that there must be boundaries somewhere and they may only be transgressed at the cost of sociocultural catastrophes. For protonormalism, the "productive chaos" of the modern age can only be restrained by a clear specification of order, which demands in particular also from the subjects a strictly conforming behavior and, if need arise, even a confirmation of those norms on which the existence of the social order is made dependent. "The protonormalist strategies," writes Jürgen Link, "invariably tend to 'lean on' a prenormalist, 'qualitative' setting of boundaries and exclusions" (Link, 1997b, p. 238). The (French) title of Foucault's famous study of the genealogy of the modern disciplinary power can be understood virtually as the motto of this authoritarian strategy: *Surveiller et Punir* (*Control and Punish*).

The flexible-normalist strategy, however, does not rely on a control from outside or even on its subjects being educated, but on their willingness to continue the self-normalization process in view of uncertain and frequently blurred boundaries of normality. "Let things happen," is their motto, occasional "excursions" ("trips") away from the center of normality into the zones of beginning deviation or even into the region of abnormality keeps society from becoming rigid. It is demanded of individuals that they offset the risk of an undesired, possibly irreversible drifting into abnormality against the opposite risk of an obsessive-compulsive orientation towards rigid and fixed norms that promise maximum security, but exhibit as their price a tendency towards self-immobilization. The flexibility of normalist subjects does not consist then in the "subjects' being permanently 'located' on the periphery," but "in an area which has a relatively large 'oscillation range,' but which oscillates around the average and for that reason remains fixed to it (e.g., sexual variability as sporadic 'outings' within the defined limits of a 'permanent relationship' or as 'serial monogamy' with different 'phase timing' etc.)" (Link, 1997a, p. 339).

What is changing during the transition to control societies is the status of the actual norm and the normalities from which the individual's position is measured. The norm no longer functions as a fixed reference for normalizing activity, but itself varies during the process of normalization; it is, paradoxically speaking, virtually the average of all deviations from a prescribed norm (regulation) imagined to be stable and resistant to time. Deviation is the normal thing. The (average) norm only exists so that deviations can continue to be recognized as deviations and they remain exposed to a gravitational force that hinders their floating around freely and uncontrolled proliferation. If it is no longer possible to establish a relation between deviation and a concept of perfection or the ideal type of nature, then at least the statistics should create a substitute for the lost social framework of reference.

We must learn to think in terms of the *immanence of the norm* (in relation to the activity that undergoes its normative influence) and also the *immanence of the resistance to the norm*. Only then will we truly stop viewing its work "as restrictive, as 'repression' cast in prohibition formulas and practiced on a subject who exists before this exertion of influence and who can free himself from such a control or be freed from it" (Macherey, 1991, p. 183). The norm does not precede its field of application, nor does it precede its own action, and this is what distinguishes it from ideals, laws, imperatives, regulations, and standards. Its normative function is only ordered to the extent that it is applied and the results of its intervention in a social field are continuously evaluated. This is why Deleuze emphasizes the variability of controls: self-forming molds that change from one moment to the next. As was explained in the beginning, statistical procedures and prognosis based on mathematical probability play a central role in this process of giving the norm a liquid character.

The self-forming molds are a precise image for the strategy of flexible normalism as defined by Jürgen Link. The norm loses its terrorist quality, which manifests itself by forcefully imposing itself upon the spontaneous will—depreciated by philosophers such as Kant as the sphere of inclination and subject to practical reason. The connection between moral concepts (guilt, conscience, obligation, sanctity of the obligation) and cruelty was revealed by Nietzsche in his *Genealogie der Moral* (*Genealogy of Morals*). These concepts, wrote Nietzsche, have "never really lost a certain savour of blood and torture," and he adds as an explanation: "not even in old Kant: the categorical imperative reeks of cruelty . . . " (Nietzsche, 1887/1913, pp. 72–73). While in Link's so-called *protonormalism* cruelty is not dispensed with and therefore the new power techniques are given the task of defending a boundary of normality that surrounds the normal field as a protective barrier if necessary, and this even possibly by force, no boundary is sacred in flexible normalism. Above all, no boundaries are set *a priori*, so that the need of having to resort to any possible means to ensure their future observance in the case of their transgression is avoided; boundaries are only set, with a bad conscience as it were, because there is a fundamental sympathy with the dynamics of modern society and its productive chaos should not be strangled by force, but only protected from irreversible effects of denormalization (abrupt breaks or antagonisms). Normalism, to modify a term of Gilles Deleuze's and Félix Guattari's, "is in a permanent state of pushing its boundary away and approaching it" (Deleuze & Guattari, 1981, p. 45), it oscillates, so to speak, equally between the spontaneous tendency towards social and cultural deinstitutionalization, or more precisely, to the largest possible expansion of the spectrum of normality and the opposite certainty that there must be a boundary somewhere. Instead of setting boundaries by authority and marking these symbolically and semantically as impermeable, flexible normalism, as it is characteristic for the control societies described by Deleuze, relies on the willingness of individuals to make the scope of their behavior an object of permanent risk evaluation.

For this reason it would be completely missing the point to associate control societies with the black utopias of permanent surveillance by "big brother" (George Orwell): Control, as Deleuze describes it, means essentially self control and refers to a certain type of subject whose style of behavior is not shaped by external guidance and education (the authoritarian character) but by self-normalization and self-adjustment.

While the protonormalists, that is, the normalists against their will, pretend in their uncertainty about the course of the boundary of normality that they are in a maximum safety zone and try to contain the fluctuations that arise from permanent denormalization and renormalization processes by definite removal of certain "minus variants" to special material territories (prison, insane asylum), a more flexible mode of dealing with the "fundamental anxiety of the modern age," that is not being normal, has been establishing itself in western societies since 1945, primarily in the United States:

> The participating subjects devise imaginary axes of normality or areas of normality with center lines, tolerance zones, boundaries of normality and zones of abnormality, in short, symbolic normalist landscapes for very different kinds of proceedings, interactions, events and processes in very different cultural sectors. They are constantly placing themselves and other subjects in such landscapes, comparing their own imagined position with that of other subjects, and determining distances between. (Link, 1997a, p. 337)

Instead of being conditioned to strictly programmed, reflex-like responses, the subjects develop the ability for self-normalization by subjecting themselves to a continuous test to find out how far they can go without toppling over the edge of the spectrum of normality and losing contact to the reassuring normality within. Deleuze hints at this aspect of a kind of flexible psycho-management that tries to guarantee the subjects' stability not at the cost of dynamics but based on them when he contrasts the "discontinuous" individual who was subjected to the disciplines, occupied a plotted space and was in this sense truly "fenced in" with the individual who is subjected to control, that is: self-control, and more likely to be "wavelike" (Deleuze, 1990b, p. 244), a quality that connotes the inevitable rolling course of this nonascertained subjectivity type who only feels sure of himself when constantly comparing his own life journey with alternative courses.

Jürgen Link shows in his *Essay on Normalism* that what he calls the "mass therapy culture" of the United States draws the most radical consequences from the principle of continuity between normality and abnormality. If there is no intrinsic, qualitative boundary that is clearly marked between normal and abnormal phenomena, then it follows that the protonormalist strategy of externalizing what is abnormal (that is, definitively separating it from normality) must be abandoned and that we have always been living in a realm that manifests both normal and abnormal aspects. The emergence of a "culture of 'therapy for the normal' " in the United States, as described by Robert and Françoise Castel in a collaboration with Anne Lovell (1982), leads consequently to a state in which there is a development of complete flexibility of all the stigmata used by a culture to distinguish between the healthy and the sick. Erving Goffman (1963), who dealt in a classic study with the contemporary forms of stigma management, shifts the perspective from normality to abnormality: how much of the abnormal is still found in what is thought to be pure normality? Not only the realm of abnormality but also that of normality has a high resolution, is differentiated, and finely graduated. What is even more significant, however, is that the differentiation within the spectrum of normality is not compact, but "flexible-continuous" (Link, 1997a, p. 80), so that in the end Goffman only speaks of "roles" in which the healthy/normal and sick/abnormal stand in opposition to each other: "One can therefore suspect that the role of normal and the role of stigmatized are parts of the same complex, cuts from the same standard cloth" (Goffman, 1963, p. 130). Stigma management is therefore "a general component of society" because in tendency there is no individual who does not participate in both roles and who is not capable of playing both roles. Goffman therefore also replaces the strict, qualitative opposition of normality and abnormality with the paradoxical "normal abnormality": "If, then, the stigmatized person is to be called a deviant, he might better be called a normal deviant" (Goffman, 1963, p. 162).

The *normal deviant* is the hero of the modern therapy culture as it was first invented in the United States—to a considerable extent under the influence of psychoanalysis, which by the turn of the century had already brought about what was considered by many contemporaries to be shocking normalization of sexual perversions. The stigma or normality management of contemporary American society now views the curing of illnesses as a "special case within an all-embracing system of 'early diagnosis' and life-accompanying normalization (readaption)." Link gives a detailed account of the institutional arrangements that lend expression to this strategy towards normalization of the abnormal or "abnormalization" of the normal as follows:

> As a result of the founding of community mental health centers under Kennedy, this trend towards flexible normalism was even given an institutional core of its own, which was followed by the tendency to transform elementary schools into de facto parallel community mental health centers (continuous testing and diagnosis of the children). A final decisive factor turned out to be the 'takeover' of Sixty-Eight (which began in the USA

> much earlier). The culture revolution (counter-culture) radically tore down the boundaries of normality (e.g. with regard to sexual minorities). The official culture then 'adopted' (as far as the legal level) some of these openings of boundaries. (Link, 1997a, p. 380)

The flexible normalism typical of control societies, as Goffman clearly illustrates, repeatedly verges on a *transnormalist realm*, a realm that functions according to the logic of free proliferation and no longer yields to the force of normalist mapping. If there is no reason to exclude abnormal or stigmatized individuals because abnormal tendencies are latently present in everyone, then it seems an obvious conclusion that the process of determining a particular positional value in the normality-abnormality continuum could be dispensed with entirely for every individual. However, precisely this consequence is not found in normalism. In flexible normalism the abandonment of permanent exclusion is compensated by constituting risk classes, whose operativeness is dependent on the individual's willingness to make self-revelations on a kind of permanent basis. The fact that this compulsion to confess can be experienced as actually pleasurable by those who are subject to it is proven by the existence of a certain type of literature, which luxuriates in biographical self-exposure and intimate confessions and supplements the active mass production of data evaluated by medical and psychiatric experts. However, the pleasure gained from revealing one's most intimate wishes (the *coming-out* effect) cannot be separated from a specific stress connected with permanent production of data pertaining to others and of that pertaining to oneself because the production of this data invariably has the function of manifesting a still acceptable, still tolerable normality, that is, with reference to the always provisional average values. "The individual is no longer confined, but indebted" (Deleuze, 1990b, p. 246). This means that he pays for his "liberation" from the horrors of abnormality by committing himself to maintaining a bookkeeping perspective towards his own small abnormalities or risk factors, which as a result must be constantly observed so that they do not develop into solid, compact abnormalities.

ILLNESS AS RISK: THE CURRENT ANXIETY

The crisis of the closed milieus, one could also say, is that their structural change, cannot be welcomed as progress or even liberation without an effort, as Deleuze shows with the example of the hospital, unless progress is generally identified with the development of more flexibility:

> In the crisis of the hospital as a closed milieu, sectoring, day hospitals or home care nursing, for example, were at first a mark of new freedoms, but then became a component of the new control mechanisms, which are not inferior in any way to the harshest confinements. There are no reasons for fear or hope, but only for seeking new weapons. (Deleuze, 1990b, p. 241)

The criterion for what Deleuze calls the "new forms of resistance against control societies" would be to avoid at all events that the fear of development of new flexibilities, which always also produce new impenetrabilities, ends up in a nostalgic perspective towards the relative security and clarity of the classic milieus of confinement. Responses to the most varied kinds of new flexibilities made possible by the normality complex of this century such as the protonormalist affect that a boundary has now irrevocably been transgressed and that "it cannot continue like this" have occurred all too often. Rather than erecting dams against the floods of permanent reforms, the willingness to resist should be made dependent on whether these reforms contain elements suitable for continuing to destigmatize the realm of pathologies or whether, on the contrary, they allow the regime of the great dichotomizations to be resurrected in a new guise.

The "new medicine which exists 'without doctor and patients' and ascertains potential patients and risk groups" cited by Deleuze (1990b, p. 247) appears at first glance to be the realization of an old dream by those who have so far been structurally underprivileged in the healing and nursing process. François Ewald (1986) has shown how the increasing penetration of the social fabric by risk technologies is also revolutionizing the conception of illness. Illnesses are now essentially "illnesses of solidarity" and are viewed according to the tuberculosis model: since "the other is a potential carrier of an evil that can strike me, it is for my own benefit that I monitor him, correct him, ensure his further development, provide for his hygiene and his sterilization" (Ewald, 1986, p. 361). Since any person can pose a risk to another, everyone is obliged to do his part in helping to reduce the risk, which means first and foremost being willing to perceive oneself as a risk. "There is risk everywhere. Germs spread, and there is the threat of their continued spread without check" (Ewald, 1986, p. 362). The paranoic eccentricities that have resulted from risk thinking introduced into our perception of illness in this century do not have to be mentioned separately. They should be a warning to us not to overestimate the human benefits of a flexible normalism. It can lead from one moment to the next to the hysteria of a general mobilization against the omnipresent evil, even in times of peace.

NURSING CONCEPTUALIZATIONS OF HEALTH AND ILLNESS

Nursing conceptualizations of health and illness, against the dichotomizing conceptualization of normal/abnormal and pathologizing of illness, emerged as a response to demedicalization of nursing in the United States beginning in the early 1970s. Within various nursing theories health and illness are conceptualized in terms of individual adaptations (Roy & Andrews, 1991), constantly fluctuating processes of experiencing and evolving in concert with the environmental changes (Rogers, 1989, Newman, 1994, and Parse, 1992), or as a continuum that bypasses the notion of normality. Such conceptualizations often maintain illness as personal experiences, not framed within the notion of "deviation from the given norm" which Foucault considers the basis for the normalizing processes of modern medicine. However, nursing work has been very much tied to the institutional base of normalizing processes remnants of the nineteenth-century hospital dynamics, which are structured around the disciplinary power of medicine. Hence, there had to exist a form of disillusion in nursing between how it proposes to conceptualize health/ illness and how it must carry on with its work within health-care institutions.

In addition, the transition to control societies from disciplinary societies that Deleuze suggests for the current scene imposes an important issue to nursing as it must shift its positioning from its earlier institutionalization within what Foucault calls "the milieu of confinement" to "open milieu." Nursing must address how it would need to conceptualize health/illness and "patient" in the context of open milieu and deinstitutionalization of control that emerges in the form of self-control and self-normalization. The conceptualization of "illness as risk" elevates the concept of health/ illness as a continuum to another level at which all is healthy/none is healthy and all is ill/none is ill. What is important for nursing is to propose how nursing as an organized system and a culture of knowledge must address deinstitutionalization of health and health care.

NOTES

1. In Bernard's work, the real identity—should one say in mechanisms or symptoms or both?—and continuity of pathological phenomena and the corresponding physiological phenomena are more a monotonous repetition than a theme (Canguilhem, 1978, p. 30).

2. A process whose counterpart is found in the simultaneously occurring installations in the schools which became a sort of apparatus of uninterrupted examination that duplicated along its entire length the operation of teaching (Foucault, 1979, p. 186).

REFERENCES

Canguilhem, G. (1978). *On the normal and the pathological* (C. R. Fawcett, Trans., & an introduction by Michel Foucault). Dordrecht, Germany: D. Reidel. (Original work published in 1966.)

Castel, R., Castel, F., & Lovell, A. (1982). *The psychiatric society* (A. Goldhammer, Trans.). New York: Columbia University Press. (Original work published in 1979.)

Deleuze, G., & Guattari, F. (1981). *Anti-Ödipus. Kapitalismus und Schizophrenie 1.* Frankfurt/Main, Germany: Suhrkamp.

Deleuze, G. (1990a). Contrôle et devenir. *Pourparlers 1972–1990* (pp. 229–239). Paris, France: Minuit.

Deleuze, G. (1990b). Post-scriptum sur les sociétés de contrôle. *Pourparlers 1972–1990* (pp. 240–247). Paris: Minuit.

Ewald, F. (1986). *L'État providence.* Paris: Grasset.

Foucault, M. (1973). *The birth of the clinic. An archaeology of medical perception* (A. M. Sheridan Smith, Trans.). London: Tavistock Publications. (Originally published in 1963.)

Foucault, M. (1979). *Discipline and punish. The birth of the prison* (A. Sheridan, Trans.). Harmondsworth: Penguin. (Originally published in 1975.)

Foucault, M. (1981). *The history of sexuality. Volume I: An Introduction.* (R. Hurley, Trans.). Harmondsworth: Penguin. (Originally published in 1976.)

Foucault, M. (1994a). Qui êtes-vous, professeur Foucault? Entretien avec P. Caruso. *Dits et écrits. 1954–1988* (Vol. 1, pp. 601–620). Paris: Gallimard.

Foucault, M. (1994b). La philosophie analytique de la politique. *Dits et écrits. 1954–1988* (Vol. 3, pp. 534–551). Paris: Gallimard.

Goffman, E. (1963). *Stigma: Notes on the management of spoiled identity.* Englewood Cliffs, NJ: Prentice-Hall.

Link, J. (1997a). *Versuch über den Normalismus. Wie Normalität produziert wird.* Opladen, Germany: Westdeutscher Verlag.

Link, J. (1997b). Von Karl Kraus zu Rainald Goetz: zwei Stadien der Medienkritik—zwei Stadien des Normalismus? In F. Balke & B. Wagner (Eds.), *Vom Nutzen und Nachteil historischer Vergleiche. Der Fall Bonn—Weimar* (pp. 235–255). Frankfurt/New York: Campus.

Luhmann, N. (1997). *Die Gesellschaft der Gesellschaft.* 2 volumes. Frankfurt/Main, Germany: Suhrkamp.

Macherey, P. (1991). Für eine Naturgeschichte der Normen. In F. Ewald & B. Waldenfels (Eds.), *Spiele der Wahrheit. Michel Foucaults Denken* (pp. 171–192). Frankfurt/Main, Germany: Suhrkamp.

Newman, M. (1994). *Health as expanding consciousness* (2nd ed.). New York: National League for Nursing.

Nietzsche, F. (1913). *The genealogy of morals: a polemic* (H. B. Samuel, Trans.) O. Levy (Ed.), *The complete works of Friedrich Nietzsche*, Vol. 13 (pp. 72–73). Edinburgh: T. N. Foulis. (Original German publication 1887.)

Nietzsche, F. (1968). *The will to power* (W. Kaufmann & R. J. Hollingdale, trans.). New York: Vintage.

Parse, R. R. (1992). Human becoming: Parse's theory of nursing. *Nursing Science Quarterly, 5,* 35042.

Roy, C., & Andrews, H. A. (1991). *The Roy adaptation model: The definitive statement.* Norwalk, CT: Appleton & Lange.

Rogers, M. E. (1989). Nursing: A science of unitary human beings. In J. Riehl-Sisca (Ed.), *Conceptual models for nursing practice* (3rd ed.) (pp. 181–188). Norwalk, CT: Appleton & Lange.

12

Nursing and Its Science in Historical Perspective*

Ingrid Kollak

This chapter places the development of modern nursing and nursing science in a historical perspective. The underlying theme is one of emancipation—the movement of both nurses and their patients from a role of subservience, first to the church, then to physicians, to one of autonomy. It is in this growth of nursing as an independent profession that the development of nursing science has flourished.

The development of nursing as a profession and science is examined by a sociohistorical method. It examines first the origins of the structures that form the foundations of our health system today as well as the differentiation that took place in the functions and roles of occupational groups working in health care system toward the end of the eighteenth century.

The history of modern clinics and other forms of health care based on the hospital system that we know today dates back to the eighteenth century. A vivid impression of the conditions prevailing at that time is given by a doctor of the period, Samuel Gottlieb Vogel, who in 1787 wrote the following concerning the famous Hôtel-Dieu in Paris:

> Here, one even sees diseases that are scarcely encountered outside their walls, which—to be sure—is not advantageous to the name of these houses of the sick. And it is only too true—alas—that the mortality in hospitals is far higher than outside them and that most of the diseases are difficult to cure in them. (Vogel, 1787, p. XXX)

*Translated from German by Gerald Nixon.

In his six-volume *Manual of Practical Medical Science for the Use of Doctors About to Practise* the critical observer and writer of these words concludes his description of the Paris hospital with the comment: "In short, a true murderer's pit!" (Vogel, 1787, XXXI).

Large hospitals like the Hôtel-Dieu in Paris, the Charité in Berlin, the Allgemeine Krankenhaus in Vienna, or the Royal Infirmary in Edinburgh were inaugurated in the eighteenth century. These hospitals, whose names have been retained for their buildings, mark a turning point in social welfare. In his study of *The Origins/Birth of The Clinic* (1975) Foucault uses the term "protoclinics" to describe the new institutions being established for the care of the sick.

To understand what is new about the protoclinics, it is helpful to give a brief account of their forerunners. These institutions were places of charity and beneficence that looked after those deprived of the care of the family and social system: orphans, the poor, the old, the sick, and the mentally ill. The primary tasks and activities of the hospitals were generally caring for the physical and spiritual well being of the inmates. Those who worked in these institutions were warders, both male and female, as well as nuns. The former lived in the hospitals with the inmates, while the nuns lived in separate convent cells. There was, however, no constant presence of doctors. In the sixteenth and seventeenth centuries a town physician (*Stadtphysikus*) was in charge of supervising the hospitals, being required by oath of office to visit the sick (Jütte, 1996, p. 41).[1]

Caring for the inmates, the organization of the daily routine of the hospitals as well as the remuneration of those who worked there all bore the stamp of the Church. Nursing, prayers, meals, and work were strictly oriented to the liturgy, the hours of the religious services determining when common prayers were said, when work was interrupted for breaks, when meals were served, and when the day began and ended. The daily lives of the nuns working in the hospitals naturally followed this rhythm, but even the kitchen workers and the cleaners, the warders, and last but not least the patients all had to adapt to the liturgical order. The chapel was the central point of the hospital and accessible to workers and patients alike. Even the meals followed the Church's calendar, with more and better food being served on religious festivals than, for example, in times of fasting.[2]

Every single person in such an institution was subjected to this strict régime. Christian love was the motivation of the carers, gratitude was expected of the cared-for, and belief in divine providence dominated ideas about health and healing. No one expected any financial reward for providing this kind of care, which not infrequently meant the life-long care of the poor. The wealthy were cared for at home and donated alms if they considered this necessary for their own salvation.

The change in the function of hospitals from providing general and nursing care for the poor to offering medical treatment was by no means a linear development. There were infirmaries that up to the nineteenth century still had the function of looking after the poor. But at the same time there were hospitals that listed in their names the groups they cared for, although these were strictly separated from each other and accommodated in different buildings. Even today the terms hospital, clinic, and infirmary are to be found alongside each other.

Characteristic of the protoclinic is a "space and language of the pathological" (Foucault, 1991, p. 9), reflected in the differentiation with regard to rooms, functions, and tasks. This differentiation made new demands on architecture as well as on the organization of patients and staff. One example of this kind of institution divided into different branches of care was the Allgemeine Krankenhaus in Vienna, opened in 1784 with over 2,000 beds and consisted of infirmary, maternity house, orphanage, infectious disease houses, and mental asylum, popularly known as the mad tower. The latter was the first institution in Europe to provide for the mentally ill (Kollak, 1997, p. 71).

Figure 12.1 is a "view of the Neue Allgemeine Krankenhaus (New General Hospital) in Vienna dedicated to all sick and women giving birth" (Kollak, 1997, p. 72). The drawing, by Petra Kleinwächter, is based on an illustration from the documentation *History of Psychiatry in Vienna* (Berner et al., 1983, p. 29).

Two things are conspicuous about this groundplan: first, it is closed to the outside and homogeneous on the inside. Second, the mental asylum lies at a distance from the main building. The whole complex has a very uniform appearance. The long rows of houses are joined and form adjacent courtyards. All the houses have two floors and, except for the gatehouses, open onto the courtyard only.

The term that Foucault uses in his book *Discipline and Punish* to describe the inner unity and outer seclusion of these institutions is that of "enclosure/seclusion" (Foucault, 1984, p. 181). Patients were systematically screened off from the outside world. The only people who had access to them were those with an authorization to enter the buildings, and doorkeepers controlled the entrances. This type of architecture was to become the standard design used in the construction of public institutions such as schools, prisons, hospitals, and barracks.

Accompanying this seclusion was an individualization in which every patient was allocated a place. In this way the many different kinds of

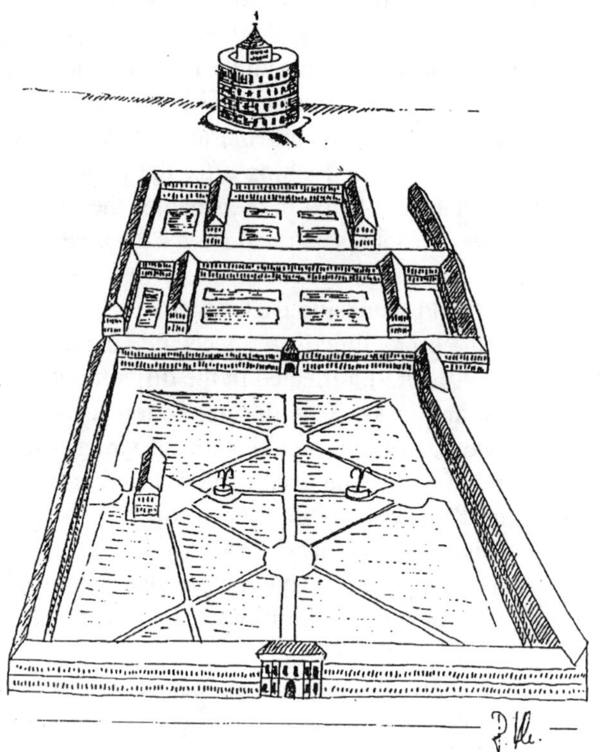

FIGURE 12.1 Allgemeine Krankenhaus in Vienna.

patients were categorized in a system in which each and every one could be located. And not only was it forbidden for the patients to leave the hospital grounds; they were also required to stay in their wards and—on the doctors' rounds, when having treatment, and at meal times—in their beds. These strict measures were also necessitated by the size of the wards, which accommodated a large number of patients in a small space.

The individualization of the patients was reinforced by the systematic registration of the patients, which subsequently took place according to numbers, the identities of each patient, and their social status, as well as their illness. The description of the symptoms, the phases of the illness, and the treatment given, along with its results, were noted and collated in patients' records, which were then stored in evergrowing medical archives. This was the beginning of a development that "took the medical documentation in hospitals beyond the stage of the occasional recording of interesting cases towards the systematic compilation of the case history of every single patient" (Jütte, 1996, p. 39).

However, locking away and individualizing the patients is only a partial description of Foucault's "art of allocation/allocating/distributing" (Foucault, 1984, p. 181). Not until differentiation took place in the functions of the new clinics, whose demands the architecture only tried to meet, did the change from the traditional hospital as part of the communal care of the poor to the clinic providing medical treatment for the sick become manifest.

From that point onward care for the poor was separated from the care of the sick. These two social obligations, both of which the hospitals had been responsible for, were now increasingly entrusted to different institutions. Thus, in the imperial state of the Habsburgs, which we know today as Austria, new laws were planned along with new administrative procedures with the aim of categorizing all those who had dropped out of society (and had traditionally made up the mixed clientele of the hospitals) and distributing them among infirmaries, orphanages, mental asylums, and houses of correction. The latter were to be attached to factories in which the inmates would have to work to earn their keep (Kollak, 1997, p. 103).

The hospitals already existing had to be restructured in accordance with these measures and had the task of identifying—out of the great numbers of inmates who had been thrown together indiscriminately—those who required medical treatment. This process can best be illustrated by taking the example of hospitals in ports. Foucault describes Rochefort, which apparently was something of a model in this respect. There, the swarms of people from all points of the compass, as well as the continual arrival of sailors with ailments and diseases of every kind, were not only treated in the port's hospital but also filtered, detained, and classified (Foucault, 1991, p. 185).

This never-ending stream of empiric material also made the protoclinics ideal places for hospital training. And this new and essential function of the new type of hospital/clinic had far-reaching effects on the evaluation of all the different work done in the clinic, the hierarchy of the staff, the organization of duties, and the role of the patient. The great variety of patients thus formed a "well-structured nosological field" (Foucault, 1991, p. 74). Diseases were studied whose carriers, the patients, were random agents. They were not interesting as subjects of their disease but as objects, whose bodies the disease had temporarily taken over (Foucault, 1991, p. 75). And this was the principle followed in carrying out examinations of the patients, where it was not so much a question of discovering diseases in the bodies of patients but, conversely, of correctly applying methods to prove the presence of a disease.

Samuel Gottlieb Vogel described the aim of his *Manual for Young Doctors* in the following terms: "My intention was chiefly to set down not only a complete, correct and faithful description and history of every disease, including its causes, but also to record as accurately as possible the traits by which it can be identified and distinguished . . . " (Vogel, 1787, p. V). The art that it was important for a doctor to master, and by which an excellent doctor could be recognized, was that of anamnesis the medical history of a patient to, according to Vogel, "penetrate into the most secret hiding-places of the disease" (Vogel, 1787, p. XXVII). Most interesting is the comparison he makes: "In short, the doctor must know how to question his patient as thoroughly as a judge interrogating the slyest of culprits" (Vogel, 1787, p. LIV–LV). Foucault speaks in this connection of a "nosological theatre" (Foucault, 1991, p. 75).[3] The fact that clinics developed into medical schools had an immediate influence on the organization of patients: besides setting up wards according to nosological fields, whereby certain diseases were grouped together, doctors began to compile files in which all their observations of diseases were noted.

Concepts of the human body as a machine *l'homme machine*, as La Mettrie wrote in 1748, or "our machine" as Mead (1759) referred to it—influenced as they were by the rise of the science of mechanics at that time—also dominated to an equal extent people's concepts of the modern clinic. Like the invisible and sophisticated machinery of the popular automatons of that period, the mechanical chess player, for example, or the mechanical musicians (Kollak, 1997, pp. 61ff), the machinery of the new clinics was expected to function smoothly, reliably, and in a purpose-oriented fashion. To keep the wheels of such complicated machinery in motion, there had to be strict organization, with people who could assert their authority to ensure that all things functioned properly. The employees needed their fixed place, their allotted task, and a working rhythm attuned to the others within this complex apparatus in order that the enormous machine called the hospital could meet the demands that its new functions imposed on it.

The "art of allocation/allocating/distributing" was soon complemented by the "supervision of duties" (Foucault, 1984, pp. 181, 192), which can clearly be seen in the protoclinics in the new time schedules that were introduced, in the definition, demarcation, and ranking of duties and, last but not least, in the role of the patients.

A vivid impression of this change in the daily work rhythm of the clinics may be gained by looking at the mental asylum at the Allgemeine Krankenhaus (general hospital) in Vienna. Doctors' visits were scheduled for the morning and evening. At this time the "mad tower" was heated in winter. The daily rhythm was then determined by the requirements of the doctors' duties such as teaching and examining and treating the patients. Around these duties all other activities were ordered. When the doctors made their rounds, the patients had to lie in bed and were not allowed to eat, for example. Nursing staff had to be at hand to undress or move the patients and to take the doctors' instructions. Medical work rhythm had replaced the daily routine determined by the Church liturgy. Moreover, the doctors were in a position to impose their time schedules on the other staff and patients. They moved into the hospitals while they were undergoing training or, if they were senior physicians, had their private studies or examination rooms there. The clinic was now centered on examination rooms and lecture theatres.

However, it was not only the daily routine that changed, based as it was on different premises. The changes in the structures and functions of the clinic were accompanied by changes in duties and responsibilities as well as in the authority and powers that were attached to these. Here the analogy with the wheels of a machine no longer fits: the wheels that revolved in the enormous machinery of the clinic did not engage automatically but by order.

The clinic had developed from a house of charitable works to a center of therapy and medical training. The work connected with the old hospitals, such as providing for the spiritual and physical needs of the poor, had faded into the background. Accordingly, the people who had been responsible for this work, the nuns and the wardens, now found that their services were devalued. The patients, too, had become unimportant as individuals; at best they were cases and at worst a hindrance to medicine when they resisted diagnosis or treatment. From a medical point of view, it was the patients' bodies that were of interest as the random and temporary homes of diseases. Similarly, the tasks that were performed in the clinics were given a critical appraisal by the doctors: tasks that had to do with the diseases themselves were given more importance, while those which had to do with the physical well-being of the patients were considered less important. As far as teaching was concerned, any work that contributed toward it was deemed useful; all other tasks were regarded as unimportant, if not obstructive.

Care for patients was henceforth divided into providing for the physical and occasionally spiritual needs of the patient by the nursing staff and the provision of medical treatment by doctors. Nursing and therapeutic treatment became two distinct fields. Wardens and nuns of humble origin carried out the former, whereas the latter was performed by doctors who had studied and who mostly came from middle- or even upper-class backgrounds. Which tasks were to be carried out when and in which way was now decided by medical directive. And for this reason doctors were soon to demand, among other things, that nursing staff should be trained to perform technical medical duties.

A society divided into classes made it possible to redefine care because an important factor in the social motivation to provide direct mutual support no longer existed. As far as care for the poor was concerned, no one spoke any longer of divine providence or the blessed poor/blessed poverty, which gave the wealthy the opportunity to do good works. Instead, poverty was now seen as having an educational function and being an incentive to work. With regard to the care of the sick, the provision of help was regulated and controlled by contract. Patients could expect help in exchange for money.[4] The classic professions such as those of doctor, priest, and lawyer were formed to help in exceptional circumstances and times of existential crisis (Luhmann, 1975, pp. 138ff). Nuns continued to work for heavenly rewards, while wardens went about their duties at all times of the day and night under the most arduous of conditions, without even being allowed to leave the wards, for a mere pittance.

There was no longer any room for either lay or self-diagnosis. On the contrary, patients were to be protected not only from themselves but also from any form of quackery; in the case of the former this took the form of strict attention to rules and control, in the case of the latter it was ensured by legally anchoring tasks and responsibilities and reserving them for the medical profession.

The accumulation of knowledge about diseases and the human body went hand in hand with the increase in doctors' authority and powers of control. This professional emancipation was achieved not only at the expense of other occupations in the clinic but also at the expense of the patients, who from then on merely had the status of objects or random carriers of the symptoms of diseases. The changes that emerged during this process had two sides to them: the separation, for example, of patients with contagious diseases from patients with noncontagious diseases was of great benefit, but the result was the registration and detention of all patients. The documentation of the progress of diseases was accompanied by the identification of the patients and by the fact that they were completely at the mercy of the doctors. There was no clear borderline between anamnesis and inquisition. Doctors' demands that nurses should be trained left no doubt who was to decide the contents of such training.

The first great wave of emancipation in health care thus did not reach everyone working in this field—nor did it reach the patients. As a result of the influence of the Enlightenment, patients were no longer regarded as being punished by divine will and their fate no longer lay only in God's hands; yet this severing of the bonds of religion meant that the place it was giving up was being taken over by medicine. Parallel to this development, however, were rising expectations of what patients, as an enlightened citizens, should do to preserve their health as well as the health of the national community.

The Art of Prolonging Human Life was the title of a book by a doctor named Christoph Wilhelm Hufeland, published in 1797, in which he gave an account of his study of macrobiotics. In his book Hufeland established a link between people's health and their physical and moral way of life. People no longer lived a life marked by predestination and subject to divine providence, but were now themselves masters of their own destiny. Well-being and prosperity were considered to be the outward expression of leading a healthy life. Increasingly, the standards for this kind of life were set by the medical profession, who, through their knowledge and authority, not only determined how the clinics were run but also attempted to an ever greater extent to exert influence on society as a whole through such matters as hygiene regulations, health authorities, or forensic medicine. Thus, besides being the controlling power in the clinic, medicine was also a "means of political intervention" (Foucault, 1993, p. 65), having a regulatory and disciplining effect for both human beings and their physical phenomena as well as for the populace and global phenomena.

It can thus be asserted that, from a historical perspective, the differentiation that took place in the domain of social care—exemplified here in the development of hospitals and occupations related to the care of the sick—was achieved without the involvement of either patients or nursing staff. Retrospectively, it can be said that there was neither a shift toward emancipation and self-responsibility on the part of the former nor an opportunity of negotiation from equal positions on the part of the latter. As far as the nursing staff was concerned, nothing more happened than a substitution of one master (medicine) for another (religion), while patients were offered nothing more than the status of being carriers of disease. Both groups were excluded, likewise, from knowledge and its acquisition and thus from the power that this brought with it in the social order.

But, what is the situation today? On the one hand it is completely different; on the other hand there are amazing similarities. The following synchronic analysis of health care inquires into this contradictory impression against the background of demographic developments, new forms of living together and changing patterns of illness. The analysis also examines the chances and possibilities that can be gained by the concept of self-care.

Help and assistance that used to be provided by social systems has now increasingly been taken over by organizations whose functions have undergone ever-greater differentiation and whose services have become more and more specialized. A concept for addressing the problem for the whole society is not at hand (Luhmann, 1975, p. 141). The path that the United States has taken is based on the concept of managed care and finds its expression in health maintenance organizations, preferred provider organizations, and capitation. In Germany there is currently a debate on the extent to which, to be able to lower ancillary wage costs, it is possible to deviate from the principle of risk share without raising the tax burden unduly and avoiding a situation in which sections of the population are left without health care.

Demographic development in Germany and the United States is currently marked by rising life expectancy with a simultaneous fall in the birth rate. Although there has been a welcomed trend toward longevity and improved health, the need for care in old age has grown dramatically in recent years. Accordingly, in many areas of the health system older persons make up the largest group of clients. Furthermore, the fall in the birth rate has led to a shift in the ratio between people in employment and those in retirement.

A shift has also taken place in the spectrum of disease. This is to be seen in the increasing incidence of chronic diseases, with circulatory disorders, malignant growths, disorders of the digestive system, and diseases of the respiratory organs leading the list of the most frequent causes of illness in Germany. The late sequelae of chronic diseases as well as relapses lead to a growing need of extensive care in old age. Added to this is the increasing number of older people in need of psychiatric care.

This development has been accompanied by a social change in forms of living together, in which the traditional family structure is in decline, while the new social units have to prove themselves in coping with situations like illness and old age. Further, women's careers as well as the increasing number of single-parent families represent a challenge to structures of caring within the family. Patients released early from hospital and in need of intensive nursing as well as those needing permanent care are looked after at home under circumstances that are fraught with difficulties. This unsettling situation affects above all the seriously ill, the old, and those living alone—not to mention their friends and relatives, who are not infrequently weighed down by the burden of care.

These developments not only represent a formidable challenge for the rigid structures of health care, which have hitherto been strictly divided from each other, but also put entirely new demands on care in the home. At the same time the occupational groups involved in health care are being entrusted with new tasks and duties. For nursing, this means not only an increase in the scope of responsibilities but also a cultivation of concepts of nursing that are oriented less toward illness and more toward sustaining the patient's resources.

For decades nurses' training in Germany has been rather one-sided, with a great degree of emphasis being put on science and technical medicine. Against this background, it is above all necessary to enrich nursing education, as rapidly as possible, with cooperative and communicative competence. The practical and technical skills and abilities, which for the most part have been well trained in the past, must now be complemented by psychosocial competence as well as being reviewed in the light of new and more flexible care settings.

Extending and increasing nurses' competence in this way is imperative to be able to ameliorate care and support both for patients and their friends and relatives; to aid them in accessing their own resources; and to harmonize what is expected by receivers of care and what is offered by care providers. Psychosocial competence is equally important in dealing with members of one's own as well as other occupational groups not only in one's own institution but also elsewhere to be able to optimize care procedures in the interests of the patients and to augment one's own achievement through effects of synergy.

In recent years there has been a rapid growth in Germany of new academic programs for nurses that bear witness to the need in our society for innovative concepts of care provision. Germany is thus catching up on a worldwide development of nursing that has been taking place for some time now. Through academic programs and the scientific grounding of nursing, the goal of emancipating nursing from medicine is now taking definite shape.

The emancipation of the patient takes different shapes in the diverse settings of the health care system. Within the walls of the clinic (or hospital) medicine rules, and it is here that medicine has its most spectacular and greatest successes. In today's world of economic pressures more and more operations are being performed on a growing number of patients in an increasingly short time. This would certainly not be possible without the support of nurses and other health care service groups that play their part in patient care. Patients who are eager to get home as quickly as possible—above all younger patients and those who can be looked after by relatives or friends—welcome their shorter stay in hospital. What is desired by patients here is speedy, short-term help in recovering health and getting back to normal life. This can be fulfilled with the help of minimally invasive surgery and day clinics as well as diagnostic and treatment centers with proper networking.

Nurses who provide medical and technical assistance will find recognition for their work as a result of their active and flexible support in the treatment of emergency cases. Those whose work contributes to the everyday running of a hospital with their untiring but less visible duties on the wards will feel that they earn too little recognition and will sometimes also feel exploited. In a clinical environment work that is related to diseases enjoys higher status than the work of catering for patients' physical and mental needs. The elderly patients and those who are chronically sick as well as those who live alone feel left to their fate if there is no reliable follow-up treatment when they are discharged from hospital.

Even today it is an established feature of the virtually undisputed organizational form of the clinic that patients neither speak out of turn nor act on their own initiative, but comply and undergo the prescribed treatment. In the clinic, patients have little or no room to influence decisions. Perhaps this will change when the self-help groups, whose members are predominantly chronically sick patients, are asked to give their assessment in the ranking of hospitals.

More room for the emancipation of the patients can be found in settings outside the clinic. People who are old or who have chronic or incurable illnesses are in need of continuing care. They enter the health care system by way of organizational forms such as outpatient care or home care. This development is in response to a differentiated need for social assistance. These more recent forms of health care organizations such as outpatient nursing or home care have the advantage for the patient that they are more convenient and not as worrying as a hospital stay in an unfamiliar environment. Patients treated in their own surroundings may feel more secure and prepared to insist on their right to be involved in decision making. On the other hand, this form of care brings with it the danger of extending the trend toward medicalization and control into the private sphere.

The concept of home care is a good example that the notion of self-care oscillates between two poles. The one pole embodies the demand for emancipation inherent in the concept of self-care, for example in the form of the patient's right to be heard, to make decisions and to be treated. The other pole embodies the normative aspect of the selfcare concept, for example in the form of the patient's personal obligation to cooperate or relatives' and friends' commitment to the family or the community.

Of equal interest is the question of the development of health promotion. There is no doubt that our society values health promotion positively. A great number of concepts have been drawn up for improving or at least maintaining the health and well-being of the population—at the workplace, in the different stages of life (for school children, senior citizens, etc.), in certain situations (for pregnancy, mourning, etc.), in cases of predisposition toward diabetes mellitus or overweight—to name but a few. A number of preventative measures are integrated into programs with financial incentives; others are tied to certain products and promoted through advertising. Not infrequently, social pressure is created by these measures, and their fiercest advocates are in favor of excluding from the health insurance system all those who refuse to subscribe to a healthy way of life—whatever this might mean in today's world. "Moral censure rests on those who do not exercise regularly and eat fast-food hamburgers for lunch" (Levine, 1990, p. 198).

Beyond moralizing appeals there is scarcely any financial or conceptual support for health promotion. The difficulties that face the concept of health promotion are illuminated in Niklas Luhmann's essay "Der medizinische Code" (1990). The sociologist Luhmann puts forward the hypothesis that the differentiation of the most important functional systems (i.e., the health care system) depends on a binary pattern that is specific to them. The examples he gives include science and its typical binary system of true/untrue, law with justice/injustice, economics with property/non-property, and medicine with healthy/sick. Although these values are related, they are not of equal value but fundamentally asymmetrical. There is a positive value like truth or property that forms the basis of action (*Anschlußfähigkeit*/ability to link with). The other value reflects the broad spectrum, the arbitrariness and the variability of the positive value (contingency). Thus, in the binary code we can find two functions: connecting and reflecting. This means that in order that research processes are initiated or that court proceedings can be held, and so forth, a positive value is required to which procedures are connected and a negative one that reflects the contingency of the former.

What is interesting about the specific functional domain of health care is that operations are connected with sick. Sick is thus the positive, healthy the negative value. A person must be sick (or at least be diagnosed as being sick) before the health care system comes into action. No one goes into hospital because they are well. That is something no one would do voluntarily. But anyone who is ill must think over very carefully how quickly he or she gets well because each bit of progress is penalized by cuts in budgets or in staff. Health facilities that encourage their long-term patients to be active and self-reliant risk financial sanctions if they let the patients make the beds. Patients who cater for themselves are seemingly an irritation to our health system and in all probability will soon be excluded from the group of those receiving care.

It is this particular feature of the health care system that explains the limited operational capacity of health promotion. Taken to the extreme in terms of the system's logic, this means that patients who are not really patients at all come together to take advantage of health promoting programs to not become patients. In other words, the health care system is taking measures to prevent people from entering the system.

The tasks of nursing are also connected with a patient's state of illness or need for care. Even the system of home care insurance (*Pflegeversicherung*) in Germany, which pays for the provision of nursing care for patients discharged from hospital or chronically ill at home, sets the amount it disburses according to the patient's degree of disability. Those who are not in need of nursing care do not receive any aid, whether financial or in the form of services, even though this might be crucial for maintaining a patient's health.

The forms of health care that a society provides have undergone differentiation and specialization. The hierarchy that has developed out of its history has largely survived in the form of clinical healthcare. Here one can still find the classic division of roles and obligations between patients, nursing staff, and doctors. The institution is focused on illness and its cure. In more recent forms of healthcare provision, however, the classic division of roles is changing. The patients' resources as well as those of their family and friends are taken into account and mobilized to a greater degree. The asymmetry that exists between nursing and the medical profession can be overcome if nursing creates a new professional domain for itself as well as a new sense of self-awareness. The emancipation of patients, on the other hand, a parallel objective of nursing science, is much more difficult to achieve. For one thing, people only become patients in situations of crisis: when they are ill, when they are restricted in their ability to lead a normal life, or when they are in need of care. For another, they never appear as a team (collective) but alone, with the sole support of relatives or friends. Nursing theories can help to define and shape society's mandate for nursing.

Finally, the diachronic study revealed that in the first emancipation of health care for nurses one master (religion) was replaced by another (medicine), while from the synchronic study it is clear that it would be a fatal mistake for nursing in its striving for emancipation to replace one master (medicine) by another (economics).

NOTES

1. Samuel Gottlieb Vogel was appointed county physician of the princedom of Ratzeburg by the Duke of Mecklenburg-Strelitz in 1780 and also county physician of the duchy of Lauenburg by the Elector of Hanover. Biographisches Lexikon hervorragender Ärzte vor 1880. Band 5. München-Berlin (Urban und Schwarzenbach) 1962.
2. In Umberto Eco's *The Name of the Rose* there is an annotation describing the organization of monastery life based on accounts handed down to us about the daily shedule of Benedictine monks. The hours of prayer determined the monks' rhythm of work, rest, meals, and sleep. The prayers included the morning *lauds* at 6 a.m., the *sext* at the sixth hour of the day (noon), and *vespers*, the evening service with Holy Communion.
3. It is interesting to note at this point that the questioning of patients that Foucault refers to, taken from Tissot's "Essai sur les études médicales," is comparable to the compilation of data that in modern nursing is subsumed under activities of daily living: breathing, pulse, temperature, thirst, appetite, digestion, senses, ability to move, sleep, pain (Foucault, 1991, p. 75).
4. In the eighteenth century, too, different classes of nursing care developed. People who could afford to pay more received better food and had their beds in different rooms from those of the very poor (cf. Stollberg, 1996, pp. 474–480).

REFERENCES

Berner, P., Spiel, W., Strotzka, H., & Wyklicky, H. (1983). *Psychiatry in Vienna. An illustrated documentation.* Vienna: Verlag Christian Brandstaetter.

Foucault, M. (1975). *The birth of the clinic* (A. M. Sheridan Smith, Trans.). New York: Vantage/Random House. (Originally published in 1963.)

Foucault, M. (1991). *Die Geburt der Klinik. Eine Archäologie des ärztlichen Blicks.* (2. Aufl.). Frankfurt, Germany: Fischer.

Foucault, M. (1993). Leben machen und sterben lassen. Zur Genealogie des Rassismus. In *Lettre Internationale* (pp. 62–67). (Übersetzung einer am College de France 1976 gehaltene Vorlesung)

Foucault, M. (1984). *Überwachen uns Strafen. Die Geburt des Gefängnisses.* (4 Aufl.). Frankfurt, Germany: Suhrkamp.

Hufeland, C. W. (1779). *Die Kunst das menschliche Leben zu verlängern.* Jena, Germany: Akademische Buchhandlung.

Jütte, R. (1996). Vom Hospital zum Krankenhaus: 16.-19. Jahrhundert. In A. Labisch, & R. Spree (Hg.), *Zur Sozialgeschichte des Allgemeinen Krankenhauses in Deutschland im 19. Jahrhundert* (pp. 31–50). New York: Campus.

Kollak, I. (1997). *Hypnose und Literatur. Der Mesmerismus und sein Einfluß auf die Literatur des 19. Jahrhunderts.* New York: Campus.

LaMettrie, J. O. (1748). *de: L'homme machine.* Paris: Gallimard.

Levine, M. E. (1990). Conservation and integrity. In M. E. Parker (Ed.), *Nursing theories in practice* (pp. 189–203). New York: NLN.

Luhmann, N. (1975). *Soziologische Aufklärung 2. Aufsätze zur Theorie der Gesellschaft* (pp. 134–149). Opladen, Germany: Westdeutscher Verlag.

Luhmann, N. (1990). *Soziologische Aufklärung 5.* Opladen, Germany: Westdeutscher Verlag.

Mead, R. (1759). *Medizinische Erinnerungen und Lehren.* Frankfurt, Germany: Brönner.

Stollberg, G. (1996). Zur Geschichte der Pflegeklassen in deutschen Krankenhäusern. In A. Labische, & R. Spree (Hg.), *Zur Sozialgeschichte des Allgemeinen Krankenhauses in Deutschland im 19. Jahrhundert* (pp. 374–400). New York: Campus.

Vogel, S. G. (1787). *Handbuch der practischen Arzneywissenschaft. Zum Gebrauch für angehende Ärzte. 1. Teil. (2. Auflage.).* Stendal, Germany: Franz und Grosse.

13

Postscript*

Ingrid Kollak and Susanne Wied

Some sciences seem to be devoid of any practice. People who learn and teach in these sciences are not infrequently questioned about the purpose and usefulness of what they do. Nursing, by contrast, is acknowledged as having a purpose and a social mission to fulfil; yet it possesses only the rudiments of science. Some people think that nursing does not have to be a science, while others actively contribute toward establishing a theory of nursing.

We assume that those who have read our book as far as this Postscript must be interested in building a science of nursing. We therefore provide neither a justification for nursing theories nor any absolute definitions of the pertinent terms because inquiry into them and discussion of them are not supposed to end with the preceding essays but are intended to be initiated by them. Neither is it our intention to make our peace with nursing theories and their terms but, on the contrary, it is to examine their contents for improvements in nursing practice, teaching, and research.

Which terms, first of all, are we talking about? We are referring to those that appear in various nursing theories but are not specific to nursing, like nursing diagnoses. We also mean terms that are familiar in everyday language, such as needs, scope, care, adaptation, and so forth. Because they are so practical and so widely and generally accepted, they are increasingly deprived of their specific meaning, even though—imperceptibly—they determine the way we think and act. The result is that to a large extent they are subjected to the personal interpretation of the reader and never subsequently questioned. We, however, insist that these terms be given a critical appraisal and considered in their proper context.

---

*Translated from German by Gerald Nixon.

In this book authors have expressed views that they currently hold about certain terms and concepts of nursing theories or about neighboring sciences against the background of their education and study as well as their experience of nursing. In various ways they have pointed out the historic and contextual significance of nursing concepts and have outlined both their possibilities and their limitations. They have done this from a diachronic point of view, by inquiring into the origin and history of a term or by examining the various contexts from which these terms are borrowed. The interpretation of these terms has always been a matter of controversy, and their meanings have undergone continual change. Of course, it is possible to introduce these terms unquestioningly into a given nursing context, but we cannot pretend that they do not have a history of their own. The authors have also presented their studies from a synchronic perspective, showing that terms are not neutral and denote a certain fact or a set of facts. Terms like interaction, adaptation, system, self-care, holism, and so forth are put into many different contexts that we cannot simply ignore. Occasionally, without any intention on our part and without us even being aware, these terms by association link us to a certain social and cultural context and its sometimes controversial implications.

Terms thus possess a dynamic of their own, a power over meaning and interpretation on which, far from being able to avoid, we are forced to take up a position. But we can also harness this power for our own ends if we learn how to handle the terms properly and use them in a creative and purposeful (i.e., knowledge enhancing) way. This book wishes to motivate its readers to indulge in theoretical reflection and enter a productive association with terms. Moreover, a prerequisite of science is unequivocal terminology, for if an object of inquiry cannot be clearly named and described, no further research step is possible.

Because our book is a co-production of American- and German-speaking authors, it may be helpful to inquire into the different conditions that exist in these countries with regard to the education and training as well as the politics of nursing.

Nursing in the United States is envied all over the world for having dealt with the question of academic and scientific status from the very beginning of this century. In Germany, as well as in Austria and Switzerland, we are still in the very early stages of such a development.

In German-speaking countries the fact that today part of the nursing profession is closely linked to Christian institutions is a result of the historic development, reflected in, among other things, the divisions in nursing federations. This is outlined in more detail in the previous chapter. The mother house system of training in the Lutheran Church, for example, functioned very efficiently up to the 1980s, but this also meant that nursing was understood as a service in Christ's name rather than a profession with special competence. The free helpers (nonregistered nurses not belonging to the deaconry, which supervised the Lutheran Church's charitable work) were instrumentalized (poorly paid with no career prospects)[1] by the leading administrators of the church training institutions (which were always headed by a pastor—never a deaconess!) in such a way as to meet existing staff requirements but not to jeopardize deaconesses' willingness to work without pay. The deaconesses' high social standing was associated with virtues such as serving, the Christian ethic of love thy neighbor, sacrifice, performing one's duty, and unconditional obedience to one's superiors—(male) doctors and clergymen. Free nursing organizations, like the Agnes Karll Federation, sprang up as a counter-movement, but they scarcely received any public attention. Nursing was instrumentalized militarily with the rise of the Red Cross, which borrowed its canon of values from those of Christian nursing associations. Under the National Socialist regime in Germany the different nursing movements were merged into a monolithic structure of fascist orientation; it took years to recover from this devastation, and the development of nursing as a profession was set back by decades.

The growing trend toward the municipal administration of hospitals forced the Christian virtues of nurses into the background. Because no new virtues came to take their place, nursing the sick turned into a relatively unspecific, auxiliary occupation in medicine without any profile of its own. The rapid achievement of academic status, which gained ground in the 1990s thanks to the untiring efforts of a number of pioneers, can do little to conceal the lack of scientifically trained personnel. Overcoming structures that are deeply rooted in history is an arduous task. And even the present generation of academically trained teachers, researchers, and managers of nursing have gone through the practical phase with all the professional conditioning connected with it.

American and Canadian nurses, on the other hand, become familiar with nursing concepts right from the beginning of their training because they study to become nurses. Study courses begin immediately after the end of high school and general knowledge learning continues in the first terms of study. Thinking conceptually about nursing, drawing concepts together with their lecturers, and evaluating them with the rest of the course is the method preferred in the profession.[2]

In German-speaking countries, by contrast, high school graduates intending to take up a nursing career are first required to enroll in a training course; this entails signing a contract with a clinic, for example, and attending the health care training school belonging to it. Here, depending on the country, they must decide from the start either in which area they wish to work in future (caring for elderly persons, children, psychiatric patients, etc.), the length of the training course, or the qualification they are aiming for. The training itself is split into two quite separate spheres as far as both institutions and personnel are concerned (although there may be close connections at the institutional level): the clinic, home for elderly persons, or other location of practical training on the one hand and the corresponding school on the other.

The clinic, with the colleagues, mentors, and supervisors (if these exist) who either work with them or are in charge of their practical training, constitutes the practical side of their training. The corresponding school, with its lecturers and tutors, provides the theoretical knowledge that is necessary. This old principle of the hospital school places the focus on the needs of the training institution and does not represent part of the general training system. It is no longer the norm, but, in Germany one can still find almost everywhere the system of lessons on one day of the week or in blocks of several weeks in which the trainees are taught by doctors, psychologists, dieticians, and nursing teachers in the individual subjects. On the other days of the week the trainees go about their work in accordance with the shift schedules of the training institution.

Should trained nurses decide to study, they can only do so after their 3- or 4-year training course (the length depending on the country) and, in addition, the required number of years' experience in health care. They then enter quite unfamiliar territory, even though their study is to be regarded as postgraduate because with excellent grades in their final examinations they would be entitled to study for a doctoral degree. At the same time, nursing concepts may be completely new to them at the beginning of their study. An understanding of nursing based on the most recent state of nursing knowledge and practice is not necessarily the starting point of nursing studies.

If we were to evaluate these different paths followed in nursing education and training with regard to their effect on kindling an awareness for theoretical reflection, we can certainly say that because of their college education American and Canadian nurses will be quite familiar with texts on nursing concepts. From the very beginning of their study they are used to inquiring into different concepts and theories so that soon they no longer overwhelm them. That nursing science is offered as a college or university course is taken for granted in the United States and Canada by teachers and students alike. All the more unconstrained, then, is the students' reception of nursing concepts, which, moreover, are not gauged purely against the standard of nursing practice. Theory and practice are two perfectly normal and equal components of training. And there lies the advantage.

Students in Germany, on the other hand, have often had to wait several years for an opportunity to study and have greater misgivings and apprehension about texts and discussions on nursing theory. These students must first learn to take a detached view of the practical experience they have gained in their previous work. If they succeed in this, they have a great advantage over others: their years of practical experience, the fact that they have mastered difficult situations in nursing as well as the task of cooperating with other professional groups and the fact that they have a precise idea and understanding of the extent to which certain theoretical concepts are valid and of how these stand in relation to the theory and practice of other disciplines.

We can thus hope in our further work together for a mutual widening of perspectives, which will ultimately have a positive effect on the development of theory as well as practice. Learning from one another can take the form of direct human exchange, as provided by student and teacher exchanges with foreign countries. Anyone who has experienced this kind of direct contact knows how inspiring and encouraging it is. And sometimes the result is to be seen in projects like this book. If similar encouragement is given to readers of this book for ideas, plans, and projects of their own, this would naturally be a great success.

From a social point of view, too, it is essential that we look further than our own back garden, as the saying goes. For as the social need for individualized forms of care grows, nurses will have to be able to integrate different, even contrary, concepts into their nursing strategies in the course of their careers. To this end, however, the pluralism of nursing concepts will also have to be taken for granted in the development of theory. (This view is not to be confused with a call for eclecticism or a system of anything goes.) Only an understanding that is emancipatory with regard to both theory and practice will be able to meet a society's need for nurses and, to achieve this, the one-sided, self-sealing view of many nurses and nursing theorists will have to broaden.

Last but not least, it is worth raising the question of the price a society is ready to pay for nursing in its practical and theoretical forms. Whereas in the United States the public funding of nursing education and research has been considerable, albeit still insufficient, the financing of nursing training and nursing research in German-speaking countries can only be described as meager. Even today, training for a career in nursing is not part of general education, and trainers at hospital schools, unlike all other teachers, do not necessarily have a university degree. With few exceptions, nursing study courses are limited to higher education colleges, and here, too, resources, both human and financial, are insubstantial. Furthermore, the development of nursing theory will depend to a very considerable extent on which projects are promoted and funded. Moreover, although winning academic status and adopting scientific standards may be great steps forward, this process must be accompanied by one of effectively raising awareness of nursing as a political issue. Here, too, theoretical concepts might variously provide a useful contribution.

The benefits of cooperation in theoretical work against the background of the different conditions prevailing in nursing practice has led us to believe that teaching and research can perhaps be summed up as follows: the common goal of our theoretical reflections on nursing is oriented toward recognizing and acting. Here, we can learn with and from each other to inquire into nursing concepts—confidently and bearing in mind the benefits to our respective fields of work—to understand which discussions and which movements these concepts are capable of sparking.

NOTES

1. Compare the confidential reports of the Kaiserswerther Verband.
2. A detailed account of nurses' education and training in the United States and the present state of nursing politics is given by Ingrid Kollak and Penny Powers in: Kollak, I. & Powers, P. (1998). *Pflege-Ausbildung im Gespräch. Ein internationaler Vergleich* [Nurses' Training under Discussion. An International Comparison] (pp. 219–237). Frankfurt/Main: Nabuse-Verlag. Written by a team of international authors, the book describes the educational, training, and working conditions of nurses in 14 countries.

Appendix

Synopsis of Selected Nursing Theorists and Conceptual Models

Hesook Suzie Kim

ABDELLAH, FAYE G.

Abdellah proposed a classificatory framework for identifying nursing problems based on her idea that nursing is basically oriented to meeting individual client's total health needs. Her major effort was to differentiate nursing from medicine and disease-orientation. Her framework identifies 21 nursing problems around which nurses must organize patient care. Although these 21 problems refer to specific aspects of patients' needs, they point to what nurses should do in meeting these needs. She did not offer specific general assumptions guiding the identification of these needs, but included among them needs associated with physical, psychological, spiritual, communicative, interpersonal, and social aspects of individual's well-being associated with health.
[Sources: Abdellah, F. G., Beland, I. L., Martin, A., & Matheney, R. V. (1960). *Patient-centered approaches to nursing.* New York: Macmillan; and Abdellah, F. G., Beland, I. L., Martin, A., & Matheney, R. V. (1973). *New directions in patient-centered nursing.* New York: Macmillan.]

HENDERSON, VIRGINIA

Henderson was one of the pioneers who tried to identify the unique contributions of nursing within the health care arena. Henderson identified 14 components of basic nursing care in association with her definition of nursing that supports the major goal of nursing as assisting individuals to gain independence in relation to the performance of activities "contributing to health or its recovery (or to peaceful death)" (Henderson, 1966, p. 15). These 14 components refer to basic human needs and everyday functioning, including bodily needs, the need for safety in relation to environment, communication, and human activities associated with worship, occupation, enjoyment of life, and continuous learning. To Henderson, nursing's role is in being substitutive, supplementary, or complementary to patients who lack "knowledge, physical strength, or the will" (Henderson, 1960, p. 7) to be independent in their daily lives. [Sources: Henderson, V. (1960). *Basic principles of nursing care.* Geneva: International Council of Nurses; Henderson, V. (1966). *The nature of nursing.* New York: Macmillan; and Henderson, V. (1991). *The nature of nursing—Reflections after 25 years.* New York: Macmillan.]

KING, IMOGENE M.

King presented a systems-oriented conceptual framework for nursing and proposed a theory of goal attainment. The conceptual framework representing knowledge essential for nursing consists of three interacting systems of the personal, the interpersonal, and the social systems, and encompasses goal, structure, function, resources, and decision making. The theory of goal attainment is the essential theoretical component of the interpersonal system within this conceptual framework. King considers the theory of goal attainment critical for nursing as interaction between clients and nurses is the essential process through which clients can be assisted to attain and/or maintain health in order to function in their roles. Several concepts are introduced in the theory of goal attainment: action, reaction, interaction, transaction, perception, judgement, role, growth and development, and goal attainment. Three specific propositions linking perceptual accuracy, role congruence, communication, transaction, goal attainment, growth and development, and satisfaction are advanced in the theory. The key to this theory is in the thinking that the outcome of nursing care is influenced by client and nurse transaction.

[Sources: King, I. M. (1971). *Toward a theory for nursing: General concepts of human behavior.* New York: Wiley; King, I. M. (1989). King's general systems framework and theory. In J. Riehl-Sisca (Ed.), *Conceptual models for nursing practice* (3rd ed.) (pp. 149–158). Norwalk, CT: Appleton & Lange; and King, I. M. (1990). *A theory for nursing: Systems, concepts, process.* Albany, NY: Delmar. (Originally published in 1981 by Wiley.)]

NEUMAN, BETTY

The Neuman Systems Model is based on the systems perspective within which clients are viewed to be open systems responding to environmental stressors in order to maintain system stability and integrity. The client system is identified by the core component of basic structure and energy resources that are protected by lines of resistance, normal line of defense, and flexible line of defense organized in a concentric circle. These lines of resistance and defense and the dynamic relationships among five variables (i.e., physiological, psychological, sociocultural, developmental, and spiritual) of the system determine how the client respond to stressors. Nursing's role is to help the client system in relation to stressors, reactions, or reconstitution in the modes of primary, secondary, and tertiary prevention.
[Sources: Neuman, B. (1998). *The Neuman systems model* (4th ed.). Norwalk, CT: Appleton & Lange.]

NEWMAN, MARGARET

Newman developed her theory of health as an expanding consciousness drawing ideas from Rogers' holistic and unitary view of humans, David Bohm's notion of implicate and explicate orders of universe, and Young's idea of the acceleration of evolution of consciousness. Newman conceptualized consciousness as pertaining to all information of a system that specifies the system's capacity to interact with its environment. Consciousness as the essence of all things that exist, including humans, is embedded within time, reflected in movement. Health as expanding consciousness is manifested in human experiences in time and space, and is expressed as transformation to more highly organized pattern of the whole. Newman proposed a hermeneutic, dialectic approach to study health and nursing aimed at pattern recognition, and a participatory research engagement that is itself a human experience of transformation.
[Sources: Newman, M. A. (1990). Newman's theory of health as praxis. *Nursing Science Quarterly, 3,* 37–41; and Newman, M. A. (1994). *Health as expanding consciousness* (2nd ed.). New York: National League for Nursing.]

OREM, DOROTHEA E.

Orem's general theory of self-care consists of three, interrelated subtheories: the theory of self-care, the self-care deficit theory, and the theory

of nursing systems. These three theories are founded upon the concept of self-care, which refers to "the practice of activities that individuals initiate and perform on their own behalf in maintaining life, health, and well-being" (Orem, 1991, p. 115). The theory of self-care is structured about the concepts of self-care agency, and three areas of self-care requisites identified as universal, developmental, and health deviation, and therapeutic self-care demand. The theory of self-care deficit identifies the connection between nursing and individuals in need of "help" due to self-care deficit. Orem delineates five modes of helping in this theory. The theory of nursing systems describes three forms of nursing systems, i.e., wholly compensatory, partly compensatory, and supportive educative systems, through which nursing agency is exercised to meet self-care requisites of patients.
[Sources: Orem, D. E. (1991). *Nursing: Concepts of practice* (4th ed.). St. Louis: Mosby.]

ORLANDO, IDA JEAN

Orlando developed her theoretical ideas about nursing based on her work related to the dynamic nurse-patient relationship, and extended them to encompass the unique contribution of nursing to patient care. She introduced four terms to categorize nurses' responses to patients needs as automatic, deliberative, disciplined professional, and nursing process disciplined. The disciplined professional and nursing process disciplined actions and reactions are viewed to be the major processes through which nurses can deliberately address patients' immediate needs by investigating patients' immediate experiences and associated thoughts, feelings and perceptions and responding to them interactively. To Orlando nursing is unique in addressing patients' immediate situational needs through communicative and interactive processes so that patients will be relieved of distress or gain greater sense of adequacy or well-being.
[Sources: Orlando, I. J. (1972). *The discipline and teaching of nursing process.* New York: G. P. Putnam's Sons; and Orlando, I. J. (1990). *The dynamic nurse-patient relationship: Function, process and principles.* New York: National League for Nursing. (Reprinted from 1961's publication by G. P. Putnam's Sons.)]

PARSE, ROSEMARY RIZZO

Parse cited Rogers' science of unitary human beings and existential phenomenology of Heidegger, Sartre, and Merleau-Ponty as providing the

core assumptions that undergird her theory of human becoming. Her theory is based on the view that humans are evolving, unitary entities in constant mutual interrelationships with the universe. Health is the expression of this evolving, experienced by humans as a process of becoming and negentropic "unfolding" characterized by meaning, rhythmicity and cotranscendence. Key concepts of the theory are imaging, valuing, languaging, revealing-concealing, enabling-limiting, connecting-separating, powering, originating, and transforming. These nine concepts are structured into three theoretical statements, which are the basis for Parse's research and practice methodology.
[Sources: Parse, R. R. (1992). Human becoming: Parse's theory of nursing. *Nursing Science Quarterly, 5,* 35–42; Parse, R. R. (Ed.). (1995). *Illuminations: The human becoming theory in practice and research.* New York: National League for Nursing; Parse, R. R. (1996). The human becoming theory: Challenges in practice and research. *Nursing Science Quarterly, 9,* 55–60; Parse, R. R. (1997). The human becoming theory: The was, is, and will be. *Nursing Science Quarterly, 10,* 32–38.]

PEPLAU, HILDEGARD E.

The focus of Peplau's theory is in interpersonal processes in nursing, especially those pertaining to relationships between patients and nurses. Her theory of interpersonal relations is generative, as she believed that encounters between patients and nurses influence the development and maturing of both participants. She identified four phases of interpersonal relations as orientation, identification, exploitation, and resolution. Within these four phases, nurses are believed to assume the roles of teacher, resource, counselor, leader, technical expert, and surrogate according to the needs of the patient during the interpersonal process. To Peplau, nursing is a "maturing force and an educative instrument" (Peplau, 1988, p. 8) and a therapeutic process that involves interpersonal relations between patients and nurses.
[Sources: Peplau, H. (1952). *Interpersonal relations in nursing.* New York: G. P. Putnam's Sons; and Peplau, H. (1988). The art and science of nursing: similarities, differences, and relations. *Nursing Science Quarterly, 1,* 8–15.]

ROGERS, MARTHA E.

Rogers' theory is based on the basic assumption that human beings are unitary beings engaged in evolutionary life processes which are unidirec-

tionally oriented and involve the mutuality with environment. The major concepts of the theory are human and environmental energy fields, which define humans and environment, and are irreducible and indivisible, signified as single-wave patterns, existing pandimensionally. Humans and their environment as energy fields are in constant, mutual interaction and interpenetrating with each other. Three principles of homeodynamics are specified as governing life processes and energy field patterns. The principle of integrality accounts for the mutual and simultaneous changes that occur in the interaction between human and environmental energy fields, and the principle of resonancy refers to dynamic, rhythmic changes in wave-patterns that accompany the mutual process of human and environmental energy fields. The principle of helicy focuses on the nature of change in energy fields through mutual processes identified as innovative, moving toward increasing complexity and diversity, rhythmic, and unpredictable. Rogers viewed her theory as a science of unitary human beings providing the foundation for developing theories in nursing.
[Sources: Rogers, M. E. (1970). *The theoretical basis of nursing.* Philadelphia: Davis; Rogers, M. E. (1989). Nursing: A science of unitary human beings. In J. Riehl-Sisca (Ed.), *Conceptual models for nursing practice* (3rd ed.) (pp. 181–188). Norwalk, CT: Appleton & Lange; Rogers, M. E. (1990). Nursing: science of unitary, irreducible, human beings: Update 1990. In E. A. M. Barrett (Ed.), *Visions of Rogers' science-based nursing* (pp. 5–11). New York: National League for Nursing; and Rogers, M. E. (1992). Nursing science and the space age. *Nursing Science Quarterly, 5,* 27–34.]

ROY, CALLISTA

The Roy Adaptation Model was developed based on key ideas in von Bertalanffy's general system theory and Helson's adaptation level theory. Roy conceptualized persons as adaptive systems, which handle inputs of stimuli, identified as focal, contextual, and residual stimuli, through two sets of control processes in relation to presenting adaptation level. Two sets of control processes are designated as regulator and cognator subsystems. Through such processing adaptive systems exhibit behavioral responses as outputs which are either adaptive or maladaptive (or ineffective). Within the model, four adaptive modes are identified as the specific areas in which adaptive responses would be observed. These are physiological, self-concept, role-function, and interdependence modes, which are oriented to specific goals for and needs of the adaptive system. Roy introduced

as an additional foundational idea for her theory the concept of veritivity, which refers to the common purposefulness of human existence.
[Sources: Roy, C. (1984). *Introduction to nursing: An adaptation model* (2nd ed.). Englewood Cliffs, NJ: Prentice-Hall; Roy, C., & Andrews, H. A. (1991). *The Roy adaptation model: The definitive statement.* Norwalk, CT: Appleton & Lange; and Roy, C., & Roberts, S. (1981). *Theory construction in nursing: An adaptation model.* Englewood Cliffs, NJ: Prentice-Hall.]

WATSON, JEAN

Watson based her theory of caring and human care on the assumption that health refers to harmony within the mind-body-spirit as a whole being and is expressed by the congruency between the perceived and experienced self. To Watson, her theory is a humanistic approach to nursing that emphasizes human to human responsiveness rooted in upholding humanistic values. Caring as the central component of nursing is oriented to health promotion and growth. Watson identified ten carative factors as the basis from which caring can be operationalized in nursing. These carative factors are the essential characteristics, attitudes, and processes through which nurses can promote health and growth in individuals.
[Sources: Watson, J. (1979). *Nursing: The philosophy and science of caring.* Boston: Little, Brown and Company; Watson, J. (1988). *Nursing: Human science and human care.* New York: National League for Nursing; Watson, J. (1988). New dimensions of human caring theory. *Nursing Science Quarterly, 1,* 175–181; and Watson, J. (1997). The theory of human caring: Retrospective and prospective. *Nursing Science Quarterly, 10,* 49–52.]

Index